STUDY GUIDE FOR BREASTFEEDING AND HUMAN LACTATION, SECOND EDITION

Kathleen G. Auerbach, PhD, IBCLC
Adjunct Professor, School of Nursing
University of British Columbia
Vancouver, BC, Canada

Jan Riordan, EdD, RN, IBCLC, FAAN
Associate Professor, School of Nursing
Wichita State University
Wichita, Kansas

JONES AND BARTLETT PUBLISHERS
Sudbury, Massachusetts
BOSTON TORONTO LONDON SINGAPORE

World Headquarters
Jones and Bartlett Publishers
40 Tall Pine Drive
Sudbury, MA 01776
978-443-5000
800-832-0034
info@jbpub.com
www.jbpub.com

Jones and Bartlett Publishers Canada
P.O. Box 19020
Toronto, ON M5S 1X1
CANADA

Jones and Bartlett Publishers International
Barb House, Barb Mews
London W6 7PA
UK

ISBN 0-7637-0829-1

Printed in the United States of America
02 01 00 99 98   10 9 8 7 6 5 4 3 2 1

TABLE OF CONTENTS

GUIDELINES FOR USING THE STUDY GUIDE

This Study Guide, which accompanies the textbook *Breastfeeding and Human Lactation,* second edition, is designed to assist both the learner and the teacher in the study of breastfeeding and lactation. For the learner, we designed this Study Guide to help assess current knowledge or prepare for certification as a lactation consultant. For the teacher, we have provided basic tools for developing a lactation course, whether it is presented with a classic academic orientation or with an emphasis on clinical skills. Additional materials for students and teachers can be found in the *Resource Guide Accompanying Breastfeeding and Human Lactation.*

This Study Guide is organized to correspond to the second edition of *Breastfeeding and Human Lactation.* Each chapter in this Study Guide contains the following:

Outline of the corresponding chapter in the textbook
- Key Concepts stressed in the corresponding chapter.

- Multiple-Choice Questions which test the learner's level of understanding of certain facts about lactation and breastfeeding. After answering these questions, the learner may compare her/his answers with the correct answers listed at the back of this book.

- Short-Answer Questions which may or may not have "one best" answer, but are designed to spark discussions among learners.

- Essay Questions which can be used for course examinations or to stimulate class discussion.

- A Story Problem which presents advanced students with a scenario requiring them to synthesize knowledge from several disciplines and to delineate actions based on this synthesis.

We recommend that the last three items be used for group work, because there is no one right answer, but rather a probable answer that depends on how each student chooses to handle the situation. These questions are ideal for inductive learning, whereby several peers participate in solving problems and thus learn from one another's experience. Because graduate study is organized for experienced practitioners to share knowledge and solve problems collectively, these last three items especially lend themselves to use in graduate-level programs.

Instructors teaching a lactation course may find the textbook too long for a one-semester course. Although each teacher will want to select chapters that meet students' learning needs and specific course objectives, we anticipate that most instructors using the textbook will choose to assign major sections of Chapters 4, 5, 6, 9, 10, 15, 16, 17, 19, and 20 for the first level of the course and the remaining chapters for the second level.

To the Students: Comments on the Study Questions

The multiple-choice questions will help you to assess your level of learning. If you select the correct answers, congratulations! You recall what you have read and are now in a better position to use that new knowledge in your daily work. If you select an incorrect answer, try to determine where you went wrong and, most importantly, why you did so. Perhaps you misread the question. Perhaps you read only a portion of the question and the options that followed, thereby selecting a "distractor" that was partially correct, but not the one best answer. Perhaps you simply didn't know the right response. If you answered incorrectly, go back and reread the question and the correct answer. Ask yourself, "Do I understand why the authors say this is "one best" answer?" If you don't understand how the correct answer relates to the question, go back to the chapter from which the question was derived and reread the portion pertaining to the question.

After you've tested your knowledge about the facts relating to breastfeeding and lactation, you'll want to go on to the short-answer and essay questions and the story problems. The short-answer and essay questions give you an opportunity to explain, in your own words, your understanding not just of the facts, but of how several pieces of information relate to one another and thus affect behavior or experience. We haven't provided answers to these questions because such answers, although based in part on the information provided in *Breastfeeding and Human Lactation*, may go beyond the material in the textbook to take into account your experiences as well. Thus, in checking your answers to the short-answer and essay questions, please refer to the textbook, but also permit a degree of latitude based on life experience and discussion with colleagues.

Likewise, when you work through the story problems, there is no one right answer, but rather a series of probable answers, depending on how you handle the situation. Make the best use of the story problems by attempting to answer each one. Don't skip a problem, such as one relating to Chapter 23 "Research and Breastfeeding", because you feel the issues don't apply to you. Each health care worker asks and answers research questions every day, every time a client presents a particular problem and you select from a variety of options a care plan that you consider optimal for that client. We recommend that you work with your colleagues when using the story problems. Perhaps one could be the focus for a journal club meeting that is reviewing a particular article or series of articles. Or, if your clinical service has a weekly meeting to discuss a particular case, ask if you might present a hypothetical case that raises issues similar to those you faced with a client; use the questions from a particular story problem to generate discussion.

Remember that when you answer the multiple-choice and short-answer questions, you are demonstrating that you know certain facts about lactation and breastfeeding. When you answer the essay questions and story problems, you are demonstrating that you can draw on that knowledge to frame responses to questions you are likely to encounter in the "real" world of lactation consulting. You will find other study suggestions in another related text by the authors, the *Resource Guide Accompanying Breastfeeding and Human Lactation*. In short, you are testing—if you use the questions provided in this Study Guide—your cognitive knowledge as well as your ability to use that information in an insightful and creative manner.

In addition to assisting learning situations, the Study Guide includes recent references that back up recommendations for breastfeeding management. It may be used for research, as it highlights questions requiring research-generated answers. It is also a guide to both current knowledge and practices in the field of lactation. (See especially the clinical implications in each chapter.)

PREPARING FOR THE CERTIFICATION EXAMINATION IN LACTATION

The certification examination in lactation/breastfeeding is designed to identify knowledge of cognitive material and the candidate's ability to use that information when confronted with problems. A certification examination requires both stamina and patience–stamina because the exam is long and patience because the actions of others, namely the administrator of the examination, will control your actions. You will do best if you enter the test situation relaxed and ready to demonstrate how much you know. To do this, you need to be able to set aside any anxieties about the testing situation. Knowing something about what you face can help reduce your anxiety. (See the box below for some general test-taking strategies.)

General Test-taking Strategies

1. Review the material over a period of time. Avoid cramming.

2. Pace yourself when taking sample examinations. Try to answer one question in one minute.

3. Read each question completely and carefully before selecting an answer.

4. Concentrate on the information offered in the question. Don't read information into the question or allow your mind to wander back to previous questions.

5. Select the one option that you think is the best response.

6. If you are unsure, eliminate clearly incorrect options before selecting from the remaining "distractors."

7. Use the answer sheet only to record the single answer you've selected for each question.

8. Use the test booklet to jot notes, eliminate options, and the like.

9. Identify the rationale for each question, and answer in terms of that rationale.

10. Use relaxation techniques if you become anxious or tense.

The certification examination sponsored by the International Board of Lactation Consultant Examiners, Inc. (IBLCE) is divided into two segments. The morning session is devoted exclusively to multiple-choice questions. The test booklet contains all the information you need to answer each question. You will be asked to record your answers on a separate answer sheet and be given a set amount of time to answer them. You may leave the examination room when you have completed this portion of the exam without incurring a penalty. Thus, if you are a quick test taker, you may have time to take a brief nap before lunch and still return to the testing site on time. If you are a slow test taker, you still should have sufficient time to complete all of the first segment of questions. Because your total score is based on the number of correct answers, it helps to made educated guesses if you don't know the correct answer. You will be allowed to write in your test booklet. Thus noting which option is clearly wrong and which ones you aren't sure of is allowed. However, make sure that your answer sheet includes only one answer for each question.

The afternoon session is reserved for answering multiple-choice questions keyed to the viewing of visual material. It is this segment that can be the most troublesome if you are unfamiliar with how such an examination is given. Practice for this portion beforehand by looking at slides or photographs and then answering imaginary questions about them. Doing this can help reduce your anxiety so that you can concentrate, rather than being distracted, by this method of testing your knowledge.

The certification examinee's goal is to pass; you need not have the top score in order to be certified. Usually the cutoff point between passing and not passing is in the mid- to low- 60th percentile (see Table 22-1 in *Breastfeeding and Human Lactation* for details). It is best to answer as many of the questions as possible. If you tend to take tests slowly, practice answering multiple-choice questions with four "distractors" within a set time limit – about one question per minute – in order to increase the speed with which you proceed through the examination. Remember, if you finish early, you can always go back over questions about which you were unsure. However, if you proceed too slowly and haven't answered all of the questions when the exam administrator asks you to close your examination booklet, you will be penalized.

Before the Exam

Using *Breastfeeding and Human Lactation* as your textbook, assign a different person or persons to lead a discussion based on a particular chapter. We recommend that all of the study group then go through the questions from the chapter being discussed. Use the multiple-choice questions as a practice session for the certification exam. Use the short-answer questions as the basis for writing additional multiple-choice questions. And use the essay questions and story problems to gain additional understanding. Setting aside a particular time each day or each week to go through sample test questions is far more effective than cramming right before the examination. Cramming doesn't help; such activity is more apt to increase anxiety by focusing your attention on what you don't know.

The night before the exam, exercise vigorously enough so that you can relax and get a good night's sleep. Go to bed early. An inadequate amount of sleep the night before reduces your alertness and your ability to think creatively in a stressful situation.

The next morning, begin the day with a meal that both provides sufficient protein and calories to keep you going for several hours and sits lightly in your stomach. This isn't the time to try out a new recipe or to include an ingredient that gave you gas three years ago! Eating a breakfast that is too light, or no breakfast at all, doesn't provide you with the energy you will need to complete the morning session.

Anxiety

If you feel panicky before or during the exam, take several deep breaths. If you know breathing techniques for labor and childbirth, use them. Close your eyes and try to visualize yourself in a safe and relaxing place. When studying for the exam, and while taking it, practice progressive relaxation by relaxing successive muscle groups. Begin with the tips of your toes and work upward, or start at the top of your head and work downward. If you feel your heart beating rapidly, tell yourself, "I'm going to breathe deeply, and my heart rate will slow." Then imagine your heart slowing as you breathe deeply and slowly several times. Some test takers say to themselves, "This is an easy exam" or "I know almost all of the answers" or "I know how to take this kind of exam." Such thoughts create a positive mindset. Avoid frightening negative messages, such as "I don't know if I can pass this test" or "I'm going to fail."

No one has expired from taking a certification exam. Ideally, you will enter the examination room alert to your surroundings and ready to concentrate on the task at hand. It's okay to feel a bit anxious, but you don't want such anxiety to interfere with your ability to demonstrate what you know. Think of the exam as a series of hurdles of varying heights, most of which will be so low that you can simply sail over them without breaking stride! Each time you answer a question, you've cleared another of those hurdles. In doing so, you will gain confidence that most of the rest of those hurdles will not cause you to trip and fall.

Multiple-Choice Questions

Most certification examinations, including the one administered by the IBLCE, consist of a long series (200 or more) of multiple-choice questions. Knowing something about this kind of question will reduce your anxiety. If you've never taken multiple-choice examinations before, you may find the structured nature of the questions difficult. Practicing with the multiple-choice questions provided in this Study Guide will help you to feel more comfortable with this form of test question.

Each question begins with a stem—either a question or the beginning of a statement—followed by four options, which are either answers to the question or the completion of the statement. Each question has one best answer mixed in with the other options or "distractors." In most cases, choices that are obviously incorrect will be easy to identify. It is your job to ferret out the one best response from among those answers that are partially correct. If you take tests quickly, you may find that the time provided for the examination is far longer than you need. If you tend to take tests slowly, you may feel rushed and frustrated that you can't set your own speed for a particular portion of the exam.

However rapidly or slowly you take tests, it is wise to practice ahead of time. Studying with peers or attending workshops designed to help candidates for certification to take "practice" exams can offer you such opportunities. Take advantage of them; simply gaining familiarity with the way questions are asked will help reduce your anxiety about being in a testing situation.

If you encounter a series of questions that are confusing—or that you simply haven't any idea how to answer—go on to the next question you <u>can</u> answer, making sure that you place your answer to that question in the correctly numbered space on your answer sheet. When you've finished the rest of the questions, you should have time to go back to the set that initially threw you.

Approach each question as if it were the only thing you cared about. Begin your assault on the question by reading it through completely. The mistake that quick test takers most often make is partially reading a question and selecting an answer on the basis of incomplete information. After you've read through the entire question, look for words that give you a clue as to incorrect distractors. Words like *always* and *never* will rarely be part of a correct answer. First identifying clearly incorrect distractors is a good way to begin if you have to guess or are eliminating certain distractors. Remember, too, that your first guess is usually the right one. Trust your intuition, best judgment, or whatever you call a hunch. However, don't hurt yourself by making wild guesses or by trying to figure out how many times item a, but not item b, will be correct.

Avoid changing answers. Very often, you will change a correct answer to an incorrect one, particularly if you are inclined to "read into" a question. It is rarely wise to try to second-guess possible writers of the question; in most cases, several individuals have contributed to each question.

Once you've completed a question, put it out of your mind. Your job now is to answer the next item. Don't dwell on a question that is bothersome or a stem that makes no sense to you. Such mulling simply wastes time that you need for the other questions. For best results, follow the guidelines in the box below.

Guidelines for Taking a Multiple-Choice Examination

1. Look for priority questions that ask for first or last actions: for example, "What would you do first?" Although all the choices offered may be correct actions, the highest-priority response is usually the <u>one best</u> answer.

2. If a lengthy situation or visual material is provided, look at the question stem first. This will give you a clue regarding what information is being sought.

3. Watch for <u>negative</u> words and prefixes; for example, "All of the following are true except." Decide on the direction of the stem (positive or negative) before proceeding with the question.

4 Select the response you best understand.

5. Trust your intuition; trust yourself. Your first hunch is usually the right answer.

6. Pace yourself. Try to complete each question within one minute. Your score will be higher if you've guessed at some questions and still finish the test rather than if you complete only a portion of the exam and all your answers are correct.

Questions Deriving from Visual Material

Long ago, Plautus (254-184 B.C.) said, "Patience is the best remedy for every trouble." Although we doubt that he was thinking about multiple-choice exams, his comment surely applies to that portion of the IBLCE-administered lactation certification exam that gives most candidates the greatest difficulty - the visual portion of the test. The speed with which you move through this segment of the exam is governed first by how well you control your anxiety and also by how much you have practiced taking an examination in this format. This section will be easier for you than you might imagine if you first identify what you are looking at, read the question pertaining to that material, decide on the best answer to the question, and then mark your answer.

Your best preparation for the certification examination is careful study coupled with creative group discussions over several months in advance of the exam. If you think of the exam as a performance, you can appreciate that regular, frequent rehearsals are the best preparation. Many successful certification candidates meet with their peers once or twice a week for several months; usually, each assumes responsibility for leading a discussion about a particular aspect of lactation or breastfeeding. The overhead/slide masters provided in the *Resource Guide Accompanying Breastfeeding and Human Lactation* will help you to present such discussions. Engaging in the student activities/projects relating to that material will also help you gain confidence.

Snacks and Medicines

Physical discomfort, such as hunger, will distract you from concentrating on the examination. If you are allowed to bring hard candies or other munchables with you, do so. When you're struggling to think through a particularly knotty question, a bit of quick energy helps you relax and enhances performance. If you're taking the examination in the middle of a sinusitis attack, a cold, or other condition, do not take a remedy that may cause drowsiness. (*Note*: The new antihistamines that most people use do not cause drowsiness.)

Sites

Examination sites differ. You may be asked to report to a hotel room, which may or may not have windows. You may be in a college or hospital classroom, a church hall, or another public space that isn't conducive to taking an exam. People who are not test takers may be making distracting noise outside the room. Lights may make the exam hard to read and the visual images difficult to see clearly. If such distractions are present, insist that your exam administrator make appropriate adjustments.

Clothing

Regardless of the season, it's best to dress in layers so that, if the room is too warm or too cold, you can remove or add outer clothing. Hotel conference rooms in the United States are notorious for being cold, almost to the point of being uninhabitable. A sweater or jacket over other clothing will keep you from being so chilled that you can't concentrate on the task at hand. Dress for comfort instead of style. Wear the type of loose, casual clothing you would choose for a day-long plane ride or car trip.

The Exam Is Over!

When you've completed the examination, celebrate having survived – and then try to forget about it. It will be many weeks before you learn how well you did. Until the day you receive your certificate identifying you as a certified lactation consultant, concentrate on the rest of your busy and fulfilling life.

SAMPLE TEST QUESTIONS

Consider these test questions in light of the techniques discussed in the preceding pages.

1. The most effective technique for using a textbook to study for an exam is to
   a. read the textbook as close to the exam date as possible.
   b. read the textbook a little at a time.
   c. write one or two questions that you think might be asked.
   d. concentrate on the summary information and the tables, if any.

- Distractor a is clearly incorrect. Following its advice is likely to increase your anxiety and prevent you from getting through the material in advance of the exam!

- Distractor b is excellent advice and the <u>one best answer</u>, particularly when you are attempting to learn and remember a large body of information – just as small meals that are well digested are more easily swallowed than large meals wolfed down.

- Distractor c is also good advice, but one or two questions are unlikely to be enough to help you remember what you've read. This answer is partially correct, but not the one best answer.

- Distractor d is good advice, but unlikely to include some of the more detailed information that you may need to know. It is partially correct, but not the one best answer.

2. When confronted by a multiple-choice question you don't understand,
   a. select the most difficult-to-understand distractor.
   b. go back to the question later.
   c. select the one option you do understand.
   d. guess at the answer any way you wish.

- Distractor a is a poor choice. The less you understand, the less likely you are to select the correct answer.

- Distractor b is a better choice. Time, relaxing a bit more, and getting into a test-taking mode may be all you need to understand the question more completely.

- Distractor c is the <u>best choice</u>. The option you understand is more likely than others to be the correct answer. Remember, the test writers are not trying to trick you.

- Distractor d is a poor choice. Guessing might be all right if you've reduced your choices down to two; this gives you at least a 50-50 chance of guessing correctly. However, guessing from four options gives you only a 25 percent chance of correctly answering the question. You will want to improve your odds before guessing by eliminating any clearly incorrect distractors.

3. When you are taking a multiple-choice test that includes visual material, how should you approach the question?
   a. Look at the picture for at least 30 seconds and then read the question.
   b. Read the stem of the question first, look at the photo, then read the options.
   c. Read the stem of the question and all of the options; then look at the photo.
   d. Look at the picture and then read the options.

- Distractor a is a poor choice. Simply looking at the picture for a long period may not tell you what is being asked. You may lose valuable time following this advice.

- Distractor b is a <u>good choice</u>. By reading the stem of the question, you may be given a clue about what to look for in the visual material. This will help you correctly select the right option.
- Distractor c is a poor choice. If you spend too much time on the written portion of the question, you may not have enough time to examine the visual material.
- Distractor d is also a poor choice. The visual material may, in the absence of awareness of the stem, give you an incorrect impression when selecting the options.

In question 3, the choices may seem less clear-cut, but there is still one best answer: distractor b. Use this technique when you practice viewing visual materials for which multiple-choice questions have been prepared.

THE HISTORICAL AND SOCIOCULTURAL CONTEXT OF INFANT FEEDING

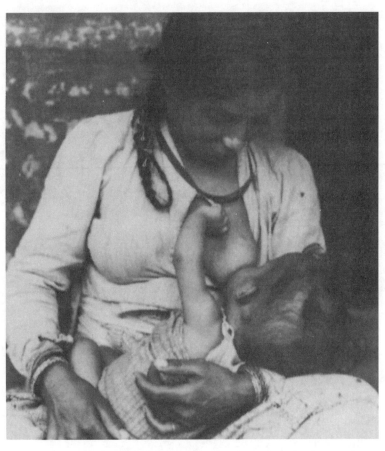

A Nepalese mother provides her baby with the best start in life. (Photo by Jack Ling/UNICEF)

TIDES IN BREASTFEEDING PRACTICE

Outline

Key Concepts

You are urged to look for these key concepts in the body of the chapter and to develop questions deriving from these concepts as one way to gain understanding and insight into their relationship to lactation and breastfeeding. You may find it helpful to compare two (or more) different cultures with which you are familiar, noting specific beliefs that influence behaviors and attitudes relating to breastfeeding and/or lactation - including its promotion and management, as well as when and how long women are expected to breastfeed.

Breastfeeding practices

Breastfeeding promotion

Breastfeeding regulation

Hand feeding

Infant mortality

Manufactured baby milks

Mixed feeds

Prelacteal feeds

Wet-nursing

WHO Code

WIC program

Multiple-Choice Questions

1. Over the last 60 years
   a. more babies are being breastfed than 60 years ago.
   b. about the same percentage of babies are being breastfed.
   c. fewer babies are being breastfed than 60 years ago.
   d. more babies are being breastfed in the developing world than 60 years ago, but fewer babies are being breastfed in the developed world.

2. Which of the following breastfeeding patterns typifies what is thought to have occurred among human groups before 10,000 B.C.?
   a. frequent breastfeeding of short duration
   b. short duration of breastfeeding
   c. infrequent breastfeeding caused by the mother's absence while gathering food
   d. frequent and extended breastfeeding

3. Giving food other than human milk to infants appears to have existed since
   a. 2000 B.C.
   b. A.D. 1000.
   c. A.D. 1500.
   d. A.D. 1850 to the present.

4. During the Industrial Revolution, high infant mortality in countries was linked to
   a. poverty among those families least likely to breastfeed.
   b. ow breastfeeding rates among those families most likely to breastfeed.
   c. high breastfeeding rates among those families most likely to breastfeed.
   d. low breastfeeding rates among those families least likely to breastfeed.

5. Giving foods other than maternal milk to infants is
   a. deeply rooted in numerous archaeological records.
   b. a very recent practice in developing countries.
   c. a very recent practice only in industrialized countries.
   d. a practice found only in people deriving from northern European cultures.

6. Using animal milks as an infant diet
   a. occurred very early in the evolutionary history of *Homo sapiens sapiens*.
   b. occurred with the development of manufacturing industrialization sites.
   c. occurred with the development of animal husbandry and agriculture.
   d. occurred only when wet-nursing fell out of favor as an alternative to maternal nursing.

7. Prelacteal feeds are
   a. an uncommon practice except in developed, highly industrialized countries.
   b. a common practice when babies are bottle-fed.
   c. an uncommon practice owing to concerns about the safety of such feeds.
   d. a common practice in many traditional societies.

8. Worldwide, infant mortality is clearly linked to
   a. poverty.
   b. a decline in breastfeeding.
   c. following Western-style feeding patterns.
   d. the advent of industrialization.

Short-Answer Questions

1. Define what the author means by "the range of 'normal' breastfeeding practices" and how that relates to current breastfeeding management. Use two examples to illustrate your understanding of "normal breastfeeding."

2. What is "wet-nursing"? Explain why, in many developed settings, it is rarely practiced today.

3. What is "hand feeding"? Identify three different forms of hand-fed foods and note their likely effect on the health and well-being of the infants who receive them.

4. Explain prelacteal feeds. Offer at least three different explanations for their use in different cultures at different time periods.

5. Explain why some investigators have concluded that, when birth is strictly regulated, breastfeeding rates decline.

6. Some writers have placed most of the blame for the use of proprietary baby milks on the drug companies that manufacture and distribute the product. Others blame physicians for attempting to replace that which nature already provides. Select which group you will defend and convince your colleagues that
   a. proprietary baby milks are a necessity in a postindustrial society. OR
   b. science can improve upon nature. OR
   c. the value of human milk is less important today than it was prior to the Industrial Revolution.
   What have you learned from this exercise?

7. What is the relationship between
   a. artificial feeding and infant health?
   b. declining infant mortality and breastfeeding rates?

8. Identify and briefly discuss four different health risks resulting from the use of artificial baby milks. Explain why some health risks appear to be short-term, whereas others are longterm.

9. Some investigators contend that, when families can afford to artificially feed an infant, it should be their choice to do so. Present a brief but clear argument showing how the cost of artificial feeding for a single family also represents costs for the community and society in which that family lives. Use one example from a developing country and one example from a developed country to support your argument.

10. What is the WHO Code, and why is it important in a developing country and in a developed country?

Essay Questions

1. The author suggests that two conditions are required for women to choose foods other than human milk for their infants: alternative foods must be available, and the use of those foods must be socially acceptable. Identify three different cultural groups.
   a. Explain what foods they use for infants.
   b. Provide examples that support the notion that those foods are acceptable for infants.
   c. Indicate the health risks and benefits derived from the use of those alternative foods within each cultural group selected.

2. Using any developed country as an example, explain how each of the following factors influences breastfeeding initiation and duration:
   a. Women's aspirations in the community and business world
   b. Women's roles relative to men's roles
   c. The availability of alternative infant foods
   d. The usual way childbirth is managed
   e. The usual way breastfeeding is managed

3. Explain the role of advertising in the distribution and selling of artificial baby milks. Give examples of three different ways in which these products are advertised - to the public and to health care professionals.

4. Identify how class differences in both a developed country and a developing country have influenced the likelihood of breastfeeding initiation and its duration. If the patterns of behavior are different, how do you explain this difference?

5. Define breastfeeding promotion and provide three different examples of how breastfeeding might be promoted.

6. Briefly review the relationship between infant feeding and
   a. inguinal hernia.
   b. urinary tract infections.
   c. otitis media.
   d. eczema.
   e. gastrointestinal infections.
   f. necrotizing enterocolitis.

   In each case, summarize the findings of at least one study that examines this relationship.

7. Explain why both the older and the younger infant are at greater risk for mortality when birth spacing is short.

8. At a local food store, price the cost of 150 cans of ready-to-feed manufactured baby milk. What does this expenditure represent for a family
   a. whose monthly income is less than $500?
   b. whose monthly income is less than $1,000?
   c. whose monthly income is at least $2,500?

   In what other ways will the use of such baby food require additional expenditures? Estimate the cost of those other expenditures.

9. Explain why duration, but not initiation, is affected by the mother's determination to breastfeed in a predominantly bottle-feeding society.

10. Explain how you would implement each of the Ten Steps to Successful Breastfeeding in a local health care facility in your community. In your explanation, note which step you would implement first, and why. Explain why you have selected the order you have for each of the subsequent steps to be accepted and how you would ensure that each is implemented.

Story Problem

You are one of a team of scientists (including an anthropologist, a geographer, a botanist, an agricultural specialist, and yourself, a specialist in infant feeding) in an area of a particular indigenous group. You must determine how the pattern of infant feeding relates to the totality of this population's way of life.

1. What are you most interested in observing before you begin to interview your subjects? Why have you selected these elements to observe, and what will they tell you?

The people you are observing use a language unfamiliar to you. You cannot get any closer than ten feet without threatening their "personal space."

2. How do you continue to gain insight into the infant feeding patterns of these people?

In the course of their own evaluations of these indigenous people, your scientific colleagues leave you near the camp to collect their own data. One afternoon, after exploring a graveyard, you sit down to rest beneath a large tree. You are wakened from your impromptu nap by a gentle tap on your wrist. You look up to find yourself staring into the deep brown eyes of a small child, who scampers back to the safety of his mother's skirt. She smiles at you and does not move away when you approach.

3. How do you let her know that you mean no harm - and that you wish to know how she feeds her children?

Two months later, your colleagues return from their wanderings, pleased to discover that you are now accepted by the indigenous group as a harmless oddity in strange dress. Prior to the scientific team's departure, each of you shares with the team what you have learned.

4. What do you tell them about the following?
   a. when mothers initiate breastfeeding, when they do not, and the duration of breastfeeding
   b. whether and for how long they breastfeed exclusively
   c. the mixed feeds that are used and how they are prepared
   d. the overall health status of the children and their mothers
   e. the role of women in the indigenous group
   f. the relationship between women's work and infant care

The Cultural Context of Breastfeeding

Outline

Key Concepts

You are urged to look for these key concepts in the body of the chapter and to develop questions deriving from these concepts as one way to gain understanding and insight into their relationship to lactation and breastfeeding. In this chapter, you are encouraged to examine your own cultural heritage in light of attitudes and beliefs that underpin breastfeeding patterns. How amenable to change are those attitudes and beliefs? And, whether or not problems arise, how might new knowledge be incorporated into the culture?

Allopathic medicine

Childbirth

Colostrum

Cultural relativism

Ethnocentrism

Food restrictions

Galactogogues

Infant care

Language

Maternal foods

Milk contamination

Religious influences

Rituals

Vegetarianism

Weaning

Wet-nursing

Multiple-Choice Questions

1. Cultural relativism refers to
   a. a belief that one's own culture is the only right way in which to live.
   b. an appreciation of one's relatives and how they live and work.
   c. recognizing that all cultures share the same values.
   d. an appreciation and acceptance of the validity of different cultural systems .

2. A ritual
   a. may involve ceremony and may reflect belief in the efficacy of a particular action.
   b. has been proven to have positive results.
   c. is usually based in nonphysiological, nonexistent elements.
   d. is derived from scientifically determined concepts.

3. In most cultures, meat
   a. plays a major role in the diet of the pregnant woman.
   b. plays a major role in the diet of the lactating woman.
   c. usually means beef.
   d. plays a minor role in the diet of the lactating woman.

4. A galactogogue refers to any
   a. clothing that covers the breasts.
   b. food believed to increase milk secretion.
   c. food believed to dry up a mother's milk.
   d. drug that alters galactose.

5. Deliberate weaning is practiced
   a. in nearly all cultures around the world.
   b. only in highly developed technological societies.
   c. only in the developing world when the mother becomes pregnant again.
   d. in those cultures where breastfeeding is considered appropriate only for a few months.

6. The hot-cold theory of foods identifies foods as "hot" when they are
   a. heated just prior to being eaten.
   b. pink, orange, or reddish in color and have a texture defined as "hot."
   c. very highly spiced, thereby tasting "hot."
   d. considered more easily digested than "cold" foods.

Short-Answer Questions

1. What is the definition of *culture?*

2. Briefly distinguish between allopathic and folk medicine. Give an example of a belief that typifies each.

3. How might knowledge of a "superfood" in a particular culture color your approach to encouraging breastfeeding?

4. In what way does language reflect cultural beliefs?

5. How might viewing breastfeeding as a process, rather than viewing breastmilk as a product, result in different attitudes?

6. For each of the following, provide an example of a positive outcome and a negative outcome, each of which helps to explain how culture influences the behavior in question:
   a. childbirth
   b. sexual relations
   c. breastfeeding
   d. wet-nursing
   e. swaddling

7. How might a 40-day (six-week) period of seclusion after childbirth assist the mother?

8. Briefly explain why "evil eye" is almost never a diagnosis offered to explain infant illness among the Alaskan Eskimos or the Aleuts of the Canadian Northwest Territories.

9. Briefly explain what is meant by complimentary proteins.

10. Briefly give several examples of food restrictions often practiced by women in different cultures during the postpartum period.

11. Identify the following foods as "hot" or "cold." Given this definition of these foods, which food would the Chinese mother be likely to eat? the Hispanic mother?

bamboo shoot	beans	beef	broccoli
cereal grains	chicken	chili peppers	fruits
dairy products	melons	soybean sprouts	oils
squash	vegetables (fresh)		

12. Distinguish between gradual, deliberate, and abrupt weaning and give an example of each.

13. Explain which and how developmental milestones are used to determine an appropriate time to wean the breastfeeding infant or child.

Essay Questions

1. Explain how culture is learned, shared, adapts to particular environmental conditions, and is dynamic. Provide an example in each case to support your explanation.

2. Using a particular culture with which you are familiar, identify a belief related to breastfeeding which is
   a. beneficial.
   b. harmless.
   c. harmful.
   d. uncertain.

3. Explain the difference between viewing breastfeeding as an assumed way of feeding instead of as a method of feeding that one is able to choose. Use at least two examples to support your distinctions.

4. Identify at least five different nonverbal messages that mothers receive regarding breastfeeding. You need not limit your answer to a single culture.

5. What is colostrum? Explain how it is viewed in different cultures and how these beliefs may influence how colostrum is used. Provide at least two examples to buttress your argument.

6. What is the "hot-cold" theory? On what is it based, and how does it influence food choices? Indicate how knowledge of this theory might be used when offering food to Hispanic women housed in a postpartum hospital ward?

7. Offer at least three reasons for weaning. In each case, indicate in what culture(s) this belief is held.

8. Select seven of the following. Identify one norm of behavior for each characteristic. Then explain how these norms might influence a woman's infant feeding choice and–if she chooses to breast-feed–how long she is likely to do so.
   a. conservative value system
   b. family orientation
   c. commitment to higher education for one's children
   d. work ethic

   e. materialism

   f. personal faith in a Supreme Being

   g. physical beauty

   h. cleanliness

   i. high technology

   j. punctuality

   k. independence

   l. free enterprise

9. Describe an alternative to a practice that is potentially harmful to the breastfeeding course or the breastfeeding mother or baby.

Story Problem

You live in a large urban city. Among your clients are women who practice the following religions: Hinduism, Islam, Judaism, Catholicism, and Presbyterianism. Among your clients are a few women who are "vegan" vegetarians and several others who are "lacto-ovo" vegetarians. About 10 percent of your clients have their babies at home; the other 90 percent give birth in three of the five largest hospitals in the city. At a prenatal breastfeeding class, dietary restrictions are discussed.

1. How would you help all 20 women feel comfortable sharing information about the dietary restrictions they have practiced or have been told they should practice?

2. Identify different restrictions that might be mentioned by one or more of your clients.

3. One of the class members asks you whether it is safe to fast, now that she is pregnant. What do you tell her?

4. Another class member tells you she "craves" foods that her religion does not allow her to eat. What do you tell her?

In the course of a home visit to a mother who gave birth 30 hours earlier, you notice that the woman's mother has prepared an aromatic drink which she wants to give to the baby as well as the new mother.

5. What do you do?

One of the mothers in your practice introduces you to her mother-in-law, who has recently arrived from Japan to help care for her daughter-in-law and the new baby. The grandmother intends to take care of the baby at night. The new father asks what he should tell his mother about bottle-feeding, since she insists that is how her "modern grandchild" should be fed at night.

6. What is your response?

7. Two weeks later, you receive a call from a mother who has been told that she should wean her baby now; she has nursed "too long." What does this mean? What do you suggest to the mother?

```
C H A P T E R
```

3

FAMILIES

Outline

Key Concepts

You are urged to look for these key concepts in the body of the chapter and to develop questions deriving from these concepts as one way to gain understanding and insight into their relationship to lactation and breastfeeding. In this chapter, you may find it helpful to compare families representing different levels of functioning from different theoretical perspectives, noting how family form and function is related to the likelihood of breastfeeding initiation and how different theoretical perspectives draw our attention to different elements within each family group.

Affiliation

Attachment

Contracting stage

Couple stage

Expanding stage

Extended family

Family functioning

Family of orientation

Family of procreation

Innovation-Decision Process

Nuclear family

Multiple-Choice Questions

1. When a second child joins a household consisting of a mother, father, and older sibling, how many relationships now exist between these four individuals?
   a. three
   b. four
   c. six
   d. ten

2. When a father has a new baby, he usually first touches the neonate with
   a. his fingertips, as he strokes the baby's arm or leg.
   b. his entire hand, as he holds the baby up for his wife to see.
   c. his fingertips, as he strokes the baby's chest.
   d. his face, when he offers a welcoming kiss.

3. According to one investigator, a family in its own adolescence
   a. has at least one teenage parent.
   b. needs a helper to point out the family's ability to cope.
   c. has only one child.
   d. is living in poverty.

4. The Innovation-Decision Process attempts to explain why some low-income women choose to breastfeed and others do not. Which of the following elements is the first step in innovative behavior?
   a. knowledge
   b. persuasion
   c. confirmation
   d. implementing the decision

5. When is a discussion of infant feeding most effective in allaying concerns and/or dispelling myths?
   a. after the baby's birth
   b. after the mother has returned home
   c. during the prenatal period
   d. after the father starts showing an interest in breastfeeding

6. Which of the following has changed more rapidly (from a societal perspective)?
   a. the conduct of mothers as mothers
   b. the conduct of fathers as fathers
   c. the expectations of others regarding the new mother's role
   d. the expectations of others regarding the new father's role

7. When is a father more likely to have a negative attitude about breastfeeding?
   a. when his previous children were breastfed
   b. when he is expecting his first child
   c. when his previous children were bottle-fed
   d. following his partner's first week as a new mother

Short-Answer Questions

1. Identify four elements considered universal to all families. Explain the importance of each element in understanding how a family functions.

2. Identify five different stages in the family life cycle. For each stage, identify when it is likely to occur and at least one problem the family must deal with at that stage.

3. Many fathers assume that father-child closeness derives primarily from feeding. Briefly explain to a class of new fathers how narrowly this assumption frames the father's role. Give at least three examples of other ways in which a father can be close to his baby.

4. Offer an example of each of the following levels of family functioning. In each case, explain how breastfeeding might be encouraged as part of the health worker's plan of care for the family members.
   a. infancy
   b. childhood
   c. adolescence
   d. adulthood

5. Using each of the following characteristics, explain why a low-income family is unlikely to breastfeed:
   a. ethnic group
   b. lack of support
   c. lack of information
   d. hospital practices
   e. hospital-based formula marketing
   f. timing of solid food introduction

6. Focusing on the same items mentioned in question 5 above, indicate how each can influence an affluent mother not to breastfeed.

7. Explain why contact with a peer counselor is likely to
   a. increase breastfeeding initiation.
   b. increase breastfeeding duration.
   c. increase time of exclusive breastfeeding.

8. Explain empowerment and how breastfeeding might contribute to such a feeling in new mothers.

9. Explain why rooming-in and breastfeeding guidance in the hospital might have a more substantial effect on breastfeeding behavior by primiparous mothers than multiparous mothers.

Essay Questions

1. A baby represents many things to a family. Briefly discuss five different reasons for having a baby. In each case, note how each reason might influence a family member's behavior toward other people, such as in-laws, friends, or colleagues.

2. Meet John. He has been a father for only three hours and has just arrived home from the hospital. On the way home, John was stopped by a policeman for weaving all over the road. Only after explaining that he and his wife had just had their first baby, following a 12-hour labor, did the policeman send him home without giving him a ticket. John knows life won't be the same. Identify for him at least three aspects of "reality" that he needs to confront so that he can make his new parenting experience as positive as possible. At least one of these aspects should deal with breastfeeding.

3. Explain why many teenage mothers prefer not to breastfeed.

4. Briefly discuss the importance of social support following a life stressor. Use three different situations involving life stress – one of which is the birth of a new baby – to provide examples of the effect of social support on different family members.

5. What is an advocate? Using an outline of words or phrases, develop a breastfeeding promotion program that takes into account the following elements:
   a. the involvement of different family members
   b. the support of key community members
   c. the receptivity of people in positions of power
   d. the resources available to those advocates for this breastfeeding promotion program

6. Explain how the following practices are related to effective breastfeeding promotion:
   a. attitude change on the part of health professionals
   b. rooming-in
   c. opportunity for early breastfeeding
   d. eliminating artificial feeding in the hospital

7. Freed examined health care professionals' levels of knowledge about breastfeeding and their confidence in being able to assist breastfeeding mothers. Briefly explain his findings relating to
   a. student nurses.
   b. family practitioners.
   c. pediatricians.
   d. obstetricians.
   e. resident physicians.
   f. the relevance of personal experience.
   g. the quality of residency/medical/nursing training.
   h. the accuracy of their knowledge of key facts about lactation and breastfeeding.

8. Examine the material on the developmental stages of families.
    a. When was Marsha's family expanding, remaining stable, contracting?
    b. In what ways were different needs required of her family at each of these developmental stages?

Story Problem

You have been hired to promote breastfeeding among the families served by a local clinic.

1. What do you need to know about these families before developing a program promoting breastfeeding?

You now know something about this clinic's population.

2. Describe it.

Taking into account the percentage of teenage families and the likelihood that some of them are composed of single women and their offspring, you present an interim plan to the clinic management.

3. Outline your interim plan.

Several of the clinic staff "talk a good game," but your observations suggest that they don't really believe that breastfeeding is all that important. At least one is actively antagonistic and is waiting for you to fail.

4. Define what that staff member means by "failure."

You believe that, if the administration backs your efforts, you will be more likely to convince others on the clinic staff that your plan is appropriate and deserves to be implemented.

5. How do you secure both the administration's active support and its financial backing?

You have set goals for yourself and for the clinic.

6. Identify the current breastfeeding initiation and duration rates among the clinic's client population.

7. Now tell us what your goals are for one, two, and three years from now.

8. How do you expect to reach those goals? Provide examples to support your answer.

ANATOMICAL AND BIOLOGICAL IMPERATIVES

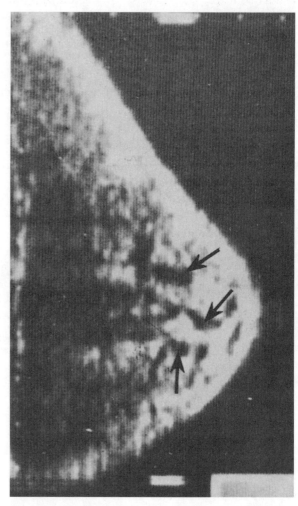

The breast. Arrows point out three milk ducts. (Thomas Jefferson University, Department of Radiology.)

ANATOMY AND PHYSIOLOGY

Outline

Key Concepts

You are urged to look for these key concepts in the body of the chapter and to develop questions deriving from these concepts as one way to gain understanding and insight into their relationship to lactation and breastfeeding. You may find it helpful to consider those hormonal and other elements specific to the lactating mother, as well as how assessment of breast and nipple tissue and infant anatomy leads to management recommendations.

Breast assessment

Breast structure

Galactorrhea

Glucocorticoids

Hormones

Human placental lactogen (HPL)

Insulin

Lactogenesis

Mammary development

Newborn oral development

Nipple function

Oxytocin

Pregnancy

Prolactin

Prolactin-inhibiting factor (PIF)

Suckling/sucking

Thyroid-stimulating hormone (TSH)

Thyrotropin-releasing hormone (TRH)

Multiple-Choice Questions

1. How does the tongue move with normal suckling at the breast?
   a. from back to front
   b. from front to back
   c. from side to side
   d. in an arrhythmic fashion so that the top of the areola is touched by the tongue throughout a feeding

2. Following birth, what happens to serum prolactin when suckling occurs?
   a. It peaks with each suckling episode, declining between feeds.
   b. It peaks with each suckling episode, remaining at peak levels between feeds.
   c. It drops to baseline and remains there.
   d. It gradually climbs over time.

3. Oxytocin secretion results in
   a. milk production.
   b. milk ejection.
   c. a sense of coolness in the mother's breasts.
   d. a heightened sense of maternal anxiety.

4. A lateral incision at _____ position is most likely to suggest severed innervation of the nipple and areola.
   a. eight o'clock on the left, four o'clock on the right
   b. five o'clock on the left, seven o'clock on the right
   c. ten o'clock on the right, two o'clock on the left
   d. nine o'clock on the right, three o'clock on the left

5. The capacity of the mammary gland to secrete milk during later pregnancy is called
    a. galactopoesis.
    b. lactogenesis II.
    c. mammogenesis.
    d. lactogenesis I.

6. As the number of mammary gland receptors for prolactin ____, breastmilk output ____.
    a. decreases, increases
    b. increases, decreases
    c. decreases, remains the same
    d. increases, increases

7. Increased skin temperature during a breastfeeding episode is a result of
    a. prolactin secretion.
    b. oxytocin secretion.
    c. cortisol secretion.
    d. TSH secretion.

8. Supplementing the breastfeeding infant will result in
    a. an increase in both prolactin and oxytocin secretion.
    b. an increase in noradrenalin secretion.
    c. a decrease in both oxytocin and prolactin.
    d. no change in oxytocin, but a decrease in prolactin.

9. The infant's tongue
    a. takes up about 25 percent of the space in his or her mouth.
    b. takes up about 50 percent of the space in his or her mouth.
    c. takes up about 75 percent of the space in his or her mouth.
    d. fills the small oral cavity of his or her mouth.

10. As milk flow _____, the rate of infant suckling _____.
    a. increases, decreases
    b. decreases, decreases
    c. increases, increases
    d. These variables are unrelated.

Short-Answer Questions

1. Briefly distinguish between suckling and sucking. During what time period does each occur?

2. Describe how you would determine that a mother has retracted nipples. What is the difference between retracted and inverted nipples?

3. What is suckling assessment, and why is it important?

4. What is meant by the phrase "obligate nose breather"? How is this related to infant feeding?

5. Marked asymmetry of the breasts may indicate what?

6. Distinguish between surgical procedures to the breast that are very likely, and less likely, to result in reduced milk production.

7. What is galactorrhea?

8. Briefly define galactopoeisis.

Essay Questions

1. Briefly discuss the notion that function changes as form changes in relation to breast size as a predictor of lactation success.

2. Describe each of the following structures and distinguish between them as to where they might be found and their function in lactation:
   a. lactiferous duct
   b. adipose cells
   c. milk glands
   d. myoepithelial cells
   e. nipple
   f. areola

3. Explain the relationship between prolactin release, oxytocin release, milk production, and milk ejection.

4. Distinguish between breastfeeding and bottle-feeding in terms of the following elements:
   a. sounds
   b. frequency of suckling
   c. breathing patterns
   d. mouth extension
   e. tongue placement and action
   f. lip flanging
   g. feeding duration

5. "What the baby does is a simple activity, involving negative pressure and swallowing what he obtains." Indicate whether you agree with this statement and, if so, why? If you disagree, how would you argue that this statement is simplistic or incorrect?

6. Explain what is meant by the "supply-demand" response.

7. Explain the relationship between breast size, milk production, and milk storage capacity.

Story Problem

You are asked to explain to a group of pregnant couples how the breast works.

1. Outline your presentation to this group.

One of the men asks,"Now I know how the breast works, but the baby has to do something, too. Right?"

2. "Right," you say. What else do you tell the group?
   The class includes two scientific types who act fascinated by the hormones of pregnancy and lactation.

3. In everyday language, explain the following and their respective roles in the lactation process:
   a. prolactin-inhibiting factor
   b. thyrotropin-releasing hormone
   c. human placental lactogen
   d. thyroid-stimulating hormone

"But, if I decide not to breastfeed," says one young woman, "I really won't be hurting myself or my baby all that much, will I?"

4. What is your response to her question?

Later that day, one of the class members calls you and asks if you can explain why she never made enough milk for her first baby. She would like to breastfeed again but is unsure if it will be possible.

5. What do you need to know about her last breastfeeding experience?

6. Indicate what she tells you when you ask questions about her last breastfeeding experience.

7. Armed with that information, what do you now tell her about her likelihood of adequate lactation with her second baby?

THE BIOLOGICAL SPECIFICITY OF BREASTMILK

Outline

Antiallergenic properties

Implications for clinical practice

Key Concepts

You are urged to look for these key concepts in the body of the chapter and to develop questions deriving from these concepts as one way to gain understanding and insight into their relationship to lactation and breastfeeding. In this chapter, you may find it helpful to consider those elements that are unique to human milk; that is, those not available in artificial baby milks or other foods given to neonates, as well as those elements that can be found in other foods. One issue to discuss is the bioavailability of those elements in human milk. Are those elements also optimally available in other foods or fluids, and what might their absence portend for short- and long-term nutritional health?

Antiallergenic properties

Antibacterial and antiviral protection

Anti-infective properties

Anti-inflammatory components

Composition of human milk

Epidermal growth factor

Hormones

Immunoglobulins

Infant growth

Milk volume

Multiple-Choice Questions

1. Human milk contains what percentage of solids to support energy and growth?
   a. 10
   b. 20
   c. 35
   d. 50

2. In most studies of milk volume, what is the approximate total volume produced by most mothers after the first month of breastfeeding a single infant?
   a. 500 ml/day
   b. 800 ml/day
   c. 1000 ml/day
   d. 1400 ml/day

3. When observing infant growth patterns over time, what pattern can be said to characterize the breastfed infant?
   a. a very early accelerated rate of gain in the first three months, followed by a slower rate of growth for the next three months
   b. a very slow rate of gain in the first three months, followed by a more rapid increase to age six months
   c. a continuously slow but steady rate of gain through the first six months
   d. no difference between breastfed and bottle-fed babies if the formula used is soy protein-based

4. When a child is not breastfed, he or she is at risk for
   a. acute illnesses, but not chronic illnesses.
   b. acute and chronic illnesses.
   c. chronic illnesses, but not acute illnesses.
   d. no statistically significant differences in likelihood of illness by feeding group.

5. The relative "maturation" of human milk is
   a. related to the number of days postpartum of the mother at the time of milk testing.
   b. related to the mother's parity.
   c. related to the frequency of feeds.
   d. currently unknown.

6. Breastfed babies need _____ than artificially fed babies to grow adequately.
   a. more kcal per body weight
   b. more calories after 5 months of age than they needed before 5 months
   c. shorter feeds per day
   d. fewer kcal per body weight

7. Milk synthesis
   a. remains stable over time.
   b. is more likely to change in multips, but not primips.
   c. can change over a period of days.
   d. can change from one feeding to the next.

8. Breastmilk storage capacity has shown that
   a. small-breasted women cannot make enough milk to adequately nourish the average infant.
   b. there is no relationship between storage capacity and 24-hour milk production.
   c. large-breasted women usually make more milk than their infant needs for adequate growth.
   d. storage capacity increases markedly only if the mother has triplets or quads.

9. Factors that predict milk intake include
   a. infant weight at birth.
   b. maternal parity.
   c. maternal age.
   d. infant weight at one month of age.

10. In order to increase the amount of fat received from breastfeeding, the baby should
    a. feed infrequently.
    b. feed only enough to reduce the mother's feeling of breast fullness.
    c. feed on both breasts at each feeding.
    d. feed frequently.

11. Lactose intolerance
    a. is more common in infants than in adults.
    b. is more common in adults than in infants.
    c. relates to the presence of lactase in the intestinal mucosa.
    d. is seen only in children who were formula-fed.

12. Pharmacological doses of vitamin B_6 have been found to
    a. enhance plasma prolactin secretion.
    b. cause neurological problems in breastfed infants.
    c. suppress neurological problems in breastfed infants.
    d. suppress breastmilk production.

13. Additional iron in the baby's diet during breastfeeding
    a. is necessary in the baby's first six months of life.
    b. will assure that the baby's iron levels remain high.
    c. will obviate the need for the mother to take extra iron.
    d. impairs the efficiency of iron absorption from breastmilk.

14. Which of the following immunoglobulins is <u>not</u> found in human milk?
    a. IgS
    b. IgG
    c. IgM
    d. IgA

15. In breastfed infants, the predominant fecal flora include
    a. bacteriods and bifidobacteria.
    b. lactobacillus and bifidobacteria.
    c. enterococci and lactobacillus.
    d. coliforms and enterococci.

Short-Answer Questions

1. When individuals refer to human milk as "white blood," to what are they referring?

2. Discuss each of the following factors in terms of its effect on milk composition and volume:
   a. the baby's expressed need for milk
   b. the mother's age
   c. the beginning of the feed
   d. the end of the feed
   e. the baby's gestational age
   f. the stage of the mother's lactation

3. It has been reported that breastfed infants consume approximately 30,000 fewer kcal than bottle-fed infants by eight months of age. Of what significance to the individual baby is this finding? Of what significance is this finding to overall infant health?

4. Briefly discuss the role of human milk in reducing infant morbidity and mortality resulting from
   a. diarrhea.
   b. gastrointestinal infections.
   c. upper respiratory infections.

5. What is the "bifidus factor," and how does it protect the breastfeeding infant's gut?

6. What is the relationship between lactoferrin and iron? Explain why exogenous iron supplements might interfere with lactoferrin.

7. Briefly discuss allergy predisposition. Note when an infant is most likely to express such a reaction, the role of genetics in determining the likelihood of allergy expression, and the role of breastfeeding in reducing its likelihood of occurrence or severity.

Essay Questions

1. For each of the elements listed below, note its primary role in nutrition of the human infant and what can occur if it is absent or present in less-than-expected amounts?
   a. fat
   b. fat-soluble vitamins
   c. iron
   d. protein
   e. water-soluble vitamins
   f. zinc

2. Briefly discuss the role of secretory IgA immunoglobulin, noting whether it is present in greater quantities in colostrum or in mature human milk. How is it thought to protect the newborn from pathogenic organisms?

3. Briefly describe the role of epidermal growth factor and its relationship to the development of the mucosal barrier.

4. Taurine has been added to some bovine-based artificial baby milks. What role does it play in human growth and development? And why was it added to at least one brand of infant formula?

5. Design a breastfeeding class presentation for expectant couples on the unique qualities of human milk and the ways in which it is a superior nutritional and health-protective fluid.

Story Problem

At the end of a three-week minicourse on human nutrition, you've been asked to present a 30 minute lecture about human milk to both first-year medical students and to students training to become physicians' assistants.

1. First, select <u>three</u> elements to call to the students' attention, recognizing that the PAs are interested in the clinical implications of what you have to say (that is, how they can use it when assisting the doctor to keep patients well), whereas the medical students are engrossed in learning all the details of everything.

After your lecture, a student raises her hand and asks, "But isn't it true that bottle-fed babies are more likely to grow better – that is, faster – than breastfed babies?"

2. How do you answer this question, focusing on both the fat volume of human milk and the total milk volume obtained in the first several months of life?

Another student stops you in the hall and asks if you will serve as a reviewer for his research project. He has decided to study iron levels in infants fed different formulas and compare them to the iron levels in infants who are breastfed.

3. What studies should he review before proceeding?

4. How might you help him with this research project?

5. List answers to at least five questions you want him to obtain in order to answer his research question.

A week after your lecture, the course administrator for a graduate class in human nutrition asks if you will meet with 15 students in a seminar focusing on allergies. They want to know about the role of human milk in preventing or reducing the severity of allergic responses.

6. Outline what you will say to this group of students, noting at least four different ways in which human milk can reduce the degree of severity of allergic responses or prevent the occurrence of allergy expression in infants.

After your presentation, several students begin talking at once. The loudest of the group challenges you: "Okay, so breastmilk reduces allergies. But what if my wife refuses to breastfeed? She thinks it's something only animals do!"

7. How do you respond to this student and to his wife's alleged reaction to your earlier recommendation to breastfeed?

Another student asks, "I can see where breastfeeding would help, particularly in the face of a family history of allergies. But what if the woman has to go back to work? She won't be able to exclusively breastfeed then, will she?"

8. How do you respond to this concern, focusing on the distinction between exclusive and partial breastfeeding, rather than on why partial breastfeeding may occur?

CHAPTER

6

DRUGS AND BREASTFEEDING

Outline

The passage of maternal drugs into breastfeeding infants

    Drug factors

    Maternal factors

    Infant factors

    Breast and milk factors

    Routes of transport

Drugs that affect milk volume

Drug safety

    Nonsteroidal antiinflammatory drugs

    Analgesics and narcotics

    Anesthetics

    Anticoagulants

    Anticonvulsants

    Antidepressants

    Antihistamines

    Antimicrobials

    Antifungals

    Bronchodilators

    Beta-blockers and antihypertensives

    Calcium channel blockers

    Contraceptives

    Diuretics

    Laxatives

    Herbs

    Scabicides and pediculicides

    Steroids

    Clinical implications

Maternal substance abuse and addiction

    Marijuana

    Cocaine

    Amphetamines

    Alcohol

    Clinical Implications

Environmental contaminants

Key Concepts

You are urged to look for these key concepts in the body of the chapter and to develop questions deriving from these concepts as one way to gain understanding and insight into their relationship to lactation and breastfeeding. In this chapter, you may find it helpful to consider three or more different classes of drugs. For each one, note its likely impact on the mother's symptoms, her milk supply, and the appearance of the drug in her milk, as well as its appearance (and in what concentrations) in the baby's serum. Additionally, for each drug considered, ask whether some other therapy can be used to alleviate the mother's symptoms – with less effect on her milk supply and/or on the baby's level of exposure to the drug in question.

Addiction

Drug diffusion

Environmental contaminants

Feeding frequency

"Guilty unless proven innocent"

Half-life

Infant age/maturity

Lipid-soluble

Water-soluble

Metabolism of a drug

Milk/plasma ratio

Molecular weight

"Phase distribution model"

Route of administration

Topical medications

Multiple-Choice Questions

1. Which of the following statements is true?
   a. Most drugs pass into human milk.
   b. Nearly all medications appear in moderate amounts in human milk.
   c. Most drugs are contraindicated in the breastfeeding mother.
   d. If administration is oral, rather than by injection, the drug is destroyed in the mother's stomach and thus does not get into the baby.

2. When is a drug taken by a mother most likely to negatively affect her fetus or infant?
   a. early in lactation, when the baby is less than one month old
   b. late in lactation, when the baby is suckling less frequently
   c. late in pregnancy, when the baby is laying down fat stores
   d. early in pregnancy, when the fetus is still developing

3. A mother is told to use fenugreek. Why?
   a. It is the least expensive item she can obtain at the drugstore.
   b. It is known to dry up mother's milk without causing pain.
   c. It is known to stop pain when applied to the skin.
   d. It is an herb, known to be a powerful galactogogue.

4. The infant will have the greatest drug exposure from breastfeeding if
   a. the medication is easily obtained.
   b. the medication is long-acting.
   c. the drug has a short half-life.
   d. the medication is protein-soluble.

5. To determine most accurately whether the breastfeeding baby has received a drug his mother is taking, measure the level of the drug in the
   a. mother's plasma.
   b. baby's plasma.
   c. mother's milk.
   d. creamy portion of the mother's milk.

6. If a mother wishes to reduce the infant's potential exposure to a medication she has been taking, when should she take the drug in question?
   a. 30 to 60 minutes before a feeding
   b. right before a feeding
   c. right after a feeding
   d. 30 to 60 minutes after a feeding

7. A baby will receive the greatest amount of maternal medication if it is administered
   a. when he is greater than three months old and taking close to 1 liter of mother's milk.
   b. when he is one to three months old and nursing at least eight times in 24 hours.
   c. when he is less than one week old, breastfeeding, and not yet stooling very frequently.
   d. when the placenta still links mother and baby.

8. All of the following are reasons why physicians are sometimes reluctant to give a breastfeeding mother a medication EXCEPT because:
   a. they assume the effects of meds on the fetus or infant are the same whether the mother is pregnant or is breastfeeding postpartum.
   b. they are not concerned with legal repercussions.
   c. weaning is an easy way to deal with the problem of whether the drug is safe for a breastfeeding mother to use.
   d. most medications pass through breastmilk.

Short-Answer Questions

1. Briefly discuss the implications of new, precise methods of measuring chemicals in maternal and infant serum and human milk.

2. Briefly discuss at least three different ways to minimize environmental contamination.

3. Identify at least six elements that can serve as guidelines for when a breastfeeding mother must take a medication. In each case, indicate how each selected element reduces the likelihood of infant exposure to the drug.

4. Explain how the infant's age affects her or his reaction to a drug the baby's mother is taking.

5. What is the effect on an infant if the mother ingests alcohol? Distinguish between small, occasional drinks and chronic or frequent use.

6. Radioactivity is an environmental contaminant with worldwide potential for serious side effects. In light of this, indicate what you would tell a mother who plans to visit the site of the Chernobyl explosion as part of a scientific investigative team. The mother has a three month-old infant who is exclusively breastfed and who will accompany her, but who will remain outside the area under investigation.

7. Explain how each of the following elements influences likelihood of passage of the drug into mother's milk.
   a. acidic level of the drug
   b. binding to protein
   c. half-life of the drug
   d. ionization of the drug
   e. lipid solubility
   f. milk/plasma ratio
   g. molecular weight of the drug

8. Explain the differences between oral, topical, intravenous, and intramuscular routes of drug administration, which is associated with the least amount of drug transfer into the mother's milk, which is associated with the greatest amount of drug transfer, and why in each case.

9. How might the mother's own health status influence drug transfer into her breastmilk?

10. Distinguish between active and passive diffusion and how each can influence the amount of drug that will pass into human milk.

11. For each of the following classes of drugs, indicate their likelihood of getting into human milk and their effect (potential or actual) on the breastfeeding infant.
    a. nonsteroidal antiinflammatories (NSAIDs)
    b. analgesics and narcotics
    c. anesthesia
    d. anticoagulants
    e. anticonvulsants
    f. antidepressants
    g. antihistamines

    h. antimicrobials

    i. antifungals

    j. bronchodilators

    k. calcium channel blockers

    l. cardiovascular drugs

    m. contraceptives

    n. diuretics

    o. laxatives

    p. herbs

    q. steroids

    r. over-the-counter (OTC) preparations

12. Some women use street drugs or controlled substances while breastfeeding. Explain the likely effects on the mother's milk supply and on the baby for each of the following "recreational" drugs:

    a. alcohol

    b. amphetamines

    c. cocaine

    d. marijuana

    e. methadone

Essay Questions

1. Explain why your concern about the effects of a sleep medication used by the mother of a newborn within 18 hours after a cesarean birth might differ if the same mother, two months later, chooses to use the same sleep medication.

2. Using the suggested questions Box 6-2, "Questions to Be Asked of Breastfeeding Mothers," role-play with a colleague who takes the mother's role. Note what other questions, if any, you might wish to ask when discussing the medication in question.

3. Identify at least three sources of information about drug use during lactation. In each case, indicate whether you would or would not use the source when seeking information about drug use during lactation. Justify your answer.

Story Problem

A mother with a two-week-old baby asks you if she should continue to take her pain pills. Although she is feeling better each day, her cesarean incision site became infected; it has since begun to heal but is still painful.

1. What do you tell this mother? Explain your rationale.

A week later, this same mother calls you and says that her nipples are reddened and extremely painful. In the course of your discussion with her, you learn that she has been taking an antibiotic since her cesarean.

2. What do you suspect may be the culprit? Why do you suspect this? What do you recommend?

Three weeks later, this mother calls to ask you if she can take the ephedrine her doctor has prescribed for her. Her asthma is back, and she needs to use her bronchodilator.

3. What do you tell the mother? Explain your rationale.

Several months later, this same mother calls to tell you that she was digging in her garden, encountered the roots of poison ivy plants, and is swollen and itchy from contact with them. Her doctor gave her a shot of Benadryl, which made her very sleepy, and instructed her to use a lotion to control her itching. She is afraid to use it, fearing that the lotion on her chest area will harm the baby if he gets it into his mouth while breastfeeding. In addition, she is afraid that the lotion will be absorbed into her skin and hence into her milk, with possible untoward effects. When she asked her doctor this question, he shrugged and suggested that she might want to wean "temporarily, or for good" now that her baby is seven months old.

4. What do you say to her about her first concern? her second concern?

5. When she asks you if it is true that her baby really doesn't gain anything any longer from breast-feeding, how do you answer her?

7

VIRUSES IN HUMAN MILK

Outline

Key Concepts

You are urged to look for these key concepts in the body of the chapter and to develop questions deriving from these concepts as one way to gain understanding and insight into their relationship to lactation and breastfeeding. In this chapter, you are asked to consider the differences among the viruses discussed, as well as their common properties. Knowledge of both will assist in making appropriate recommendations to clients and other health care workers.

Chickenpox (Herpes zoster)

Cytomegalovirus

Hepatitis B

Herpes simplex

Human immunodeficiency virus (HIV)

Passive immunity

Retrovirus

Rubella

Seroconversion

Viral transmission

Multiple-Choice Questions

1. Universal precautions designed to protect health workers against infection through contact with patients apply to all of the following EXCEPT
   a. blood.
   b. human milk.
   c. semen.
   d. vaginal secretions.

2. Which of the following viruses is most prevalent in the adult population?
   a. herpes simplex
   b. hepatitis B
   c. rubella
   d. cytomegalovirus

3. Which of the following viruses contraindicates breastfeeding?
   a. rubella
   b. hepatitis B
   c. HTLV-1
   d. herpes simplex

4. The human immunovirus is one of a class of _____ viruses.
   a. envelope
   b. package
   c. intercellular
   d. low specificity

5. When a baby is born to a mother infected with HIV, the risk of transmission of the virus through breastfeeding is
   a. effectively nullified from the previous transmission and potential infection rate.
   b. greater than 50 percent.
   c. estimated to be 8 to 18 percent greater than the fetal transmission rate.
   d. highest in women in industrialized settings.

6. Which of the following factors does NOT increase the risk of HIV vertical transmission?
   a. immune deficiency in the mother
   b. low CD4+ lymphocyte count
   c. premature rupture of the membranes
   d. short-term (less than eight months) breastfeeding

7. When is HSV infection most likely to be serious in the infant of the mother who is HSV positive?
   a. when the child is nearly one year of age
   b. when the child is newborn
   c. when the child is more than one month but less than six months old
   d. Age has nothing to do with the seriousness of this infection.

8. Assuming the newborn receives passive immunity from childhood diseases from the mother, about how long will this immunity last?
   a. three to six months
   b. two months
   c. one month
   d. one week

Short-Answer Questions

1. Distinguish between intracellular and intercellular as they relate to viruses and how they may be transmitted.

2. What is an enveloped virus?

3. Under what circumstances might a mother with herpes zoster continue to breastfeed her infant?

4. Explain why rubella causes birth defects, but is not a cause for concern if it is found in human milk.

5. How might the incidence of hepatitis B infection be reduced in neonates, according to one study reported in this chapter? How is breastfeeding related to neonatal infection rates?

6. "The concern of health providers should be directed at mothers who have an unidentified infection." What is meant by this statement? How is it related to the infant feeding method the mother has chosen?

7. Briefly explain the term *passive immunity.*

8. Under what circumstances, for viruses other than HIV, should a mother not breastfeed?

9. Explain how zidovudine and protease inhibitors are thought to reduce the risk of vertical transmission of HIV.

10. Describe how the timing of infection with HIV is related to risk of transmission to the fetus/infant. Identify when the risk of transmission is lowest and when it is highest.

Essay Questions

1. Develop a chart that includes the following information in its headings: route(s) of transmission, the likelihood of infection in the neonate, whether the infection is acute or chronic, and means of preventing cross-contamination. Complete the chart by filling in information under every heading for each of the following viruses: herpes simplex, cytomegalovirus, herpes zoster, hepatitis B, hepatitis C, HTLV-1, and rubella. When your chart is complete, evaluate the similarities among these viruses, In what ways do they differ?

2. Explain why the author of this chapter concludes that a viral infection in the mother is "rarely" a reason for terminating breastfeeding.

3. Develop a brief (one-page) statement designed to inform its readers of your views on the advisability of breastfeeding when the mother of a neonate has a viral infection. Include comments about the risk of breastfeeding an older child when the mother has a viral infection. Include examples relating to at least four different viruses in support of your policy statement.

4. Discuss the differences in recommendations relating to whether a woman should breastfeed if she is HIV positive and how this relates to women (a) in developed countries and (b) in developing countries.

5. Compare hepatitis B and hepatitis C with regard to the following:
   a. likelihood of transmission to the fetus
   b. likelihood of transmission through breastfeeding
   c. recommendations relating to continuation/termination of breastfeeding
   d. potential for protection of the child later in life
   e. potential for later chronic illnesses as a result of exposure to the virus as a fetus or newborn

Story Problem

You are asked to assist a mother who has expressed a desire to breastfeed. However, the herpes infection she has harbored since she was 20 years old became active shortly before she went into labor.

1. What do you tell her about her illness?

2. What do you tell her about the desirability of breastfeeding this baby?

This mother's baby is rooming in with her throughout her entire hospital stay.

3. What do you tell this mother in order to help her see how beneficial such 24-hour rooming-in will be?

A mother is housed in the room farthest from the newborn nursery. Her baby was stillborn, and the mother tested positive for HIV. You are asked to help this mother because she is complaining of breast engorgement.

4. What kind of precautions do you take before entering her room? while helping her?

5. How do you answer her implied question that her HIV status was what "killed my baby"?

A mother calls you two months after her baby's birth. She has contracted chickenpox after having been exposed to the disease through her five-year-old child.

6. What is your reply to her concerns about her breastfeeding baby's risk of contracting chickenpox?

PRENATAL, PERINATAL, AND POSTNATAL PERIODS

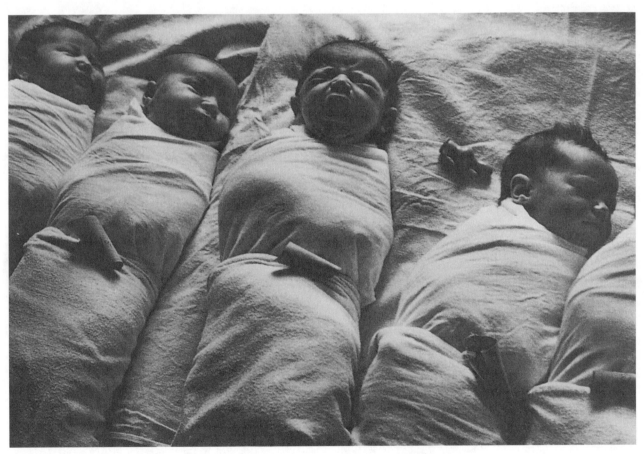

While babies share many common virtues, each is an individual. (Photo by Sergei Vasiliev)

C H A P T E R

8

BREASTFEEDING EDUCATION

Outline

Learning principles

Adult education

Curriculum development

The change process

Parent education

    Prenatal education

    Early breastfeeding education

    Continuing support for breastfeeding families

How effective is breastfeeding education?

Teaching strategies

Therapeutic communication

Small group dynamics

Multimedia presentations

    Slides

    Transparencies

    Videotapes

    CD ROMs

Educational materials

Education for at-risk populations

Educational needs and early discharge

Health care provider education

    Continuing education

    Objectives and outcomes

The team approach

Lactation Consultants

Key Concepts

You are urged to look for these key concepts in the body of the chapter and to develop questions deriving from these concepts as one way to gain understanding and insight into their relationship to lactation and breastfeeding. In this chapter, you are asked to consider the many ways in which expertise with lactation can be acquired, and the benefits and limitations of each option. In what ways do these options for professional lactation education mirror the educational resources for other health care providers? Additionally you may find it useful to evaluate local opportunities available for women to become informed about optimal infant feeding, and to see how such opportunities serve as an alternative to commercially advertised artificial feeding methods.

Adult education

Breastfeeding education

Change process

Continuing education

Curriculum development

Infant feeding decision

Learner objectives

Learning principles

Parent education

Practical information

Small group dynamics

Teaching strategies

Team approach

Therapeutic communication

Multiple-Choice Questions

1. Adult learners differ from children in which of the following ways?
   a. adults are other-directed
   b. time is considered the least valuable of all adult assets
   c. education must include the theoretical underpinnings of action
   d. education must be applicable to real life

2. All but ONE of the following purposes are common to breastfeeding education programs.
   a. to provide neutral information about infant feeding
   b. to provide practical information about breastfeeding
   c. to provide ongoing support for women choosing to breastfeed
   d. to provide encouragement to women who might not otherwise breastfeed

3. For optimal learning and change in behavior, the ideal group size ranges from
   a. 1 to 5 persons.
   b. 3 to 7 persons.
   c. 8 to 12 persons.
   d. 13 to 24 persons.

4. The utilization model of curriculum development focuses on
   a. presenting information in the order of its usual occurrence.
   b. presenting information when participants most need it.
   c. moving from the simple to the complex when presenting information.
   d. moving from the known to the unknown when presenting information.

5. A teachable moment refers to a time when a learner
   a. takes over for the teacher to make a point.
   b. passes a test question.
   c. perceives a personal need for new information or skills.
   d. registers for a distance learning course.

6. Kinesthetic learning occurs when the learner
   a. touches or handles material referred to in the lesson.
   b. hears material, as when attending a lecture.
   c. reads new information.
   d. uses as many senses as possible to incorporate new knowledge.

7. The most effective learning occurs when the learner
   a. touches or handles material referred to in the lesson.
   b. hears material, as when attending a lecture.
   c. reads new information.
   d. uses as many senses as possible to incorporate new knowledge.

Short-Answer Questions

1. What is a teachable moment?

2. Distinguish among auditory, kinesthetic, and visual learning. How might breastfeeding skills be taught using each of these techniques?

3. For each of the stages of acquisition of parenthood, identify two elements of learning that new parents should master.

4. Select at least five items about which breastfeeding mothers need information. Provide one or two sentences of information about each item.

5. What is therapeutic communication?

6. Briefly identify at least three characteristics of effective educational materials.

7. What is continuing education?

8. Briefly explain how each of the following elements can limit the effectiveness of an educational program designed for health care providers:
   a. participants' lack of confidence
   b. participants' sensitivity to failure
   c. participants' poor self-concept
   d. participants' resistance to change

9. What is a change agent?

10. Briefly explain how a telephone warmline might be used to generate greater staff support for a more extensive program of breastfeeding education and support.

Essay Questions

1. The authors suggest that breastfeeding education involves cognitive skills, affective learning, and psychomotor skills. Briefly identify elements of breastfeeding education within each category, and provide an example of each for women wanting to learn how to breastfeed and for health care workers for whom knowledge of the lactation course is seen as appropriate to their area of specialization or practice.

2. Select a specific topic pertaining to breastfeeding. Outline your teaching session, making clear its introduction, learning experience, and conclusion or summary.

3. "Supplying information about breastfeeding management is sufficient to assure breastfeeding success." Debate the merits of this statement by providing at least two examples to support your contention that the statement is true and two examples of why the statement is false.

4. Indicate how each of the following team members might contribute to a medical center's breastfeeding education program for health care providers:
   a. perinatal nurses
   b. childbirth educators
   c. dietitians
   d. lactation consultants
   e. community-based volunteer support groups
   f. physicians

5. Identify one aspect of a hospital or clinic setting that you wish to change as it relates to breastfeeding promotion, protection, or support. Outline how you would plan for that change, noting where resistance is most likely to come from and how you will counter such resistance.

6. Briefly describe and give an example of each of the following models for organizing a teaching curriculum:
   a. the chronological model
   b. the utilization model
   c. moving from simple to complex
   d. moving from general to specific
   e. moving from known to unknown

7. Review the different processes for enabling change. Select an example of a change, and identify how it might move through the steps in the change process.

8. Review the six modifiable variables that predict breastfeeding outcome. For each of the maternal-related items, discuss how each variable might influence a mother's actions. For each of the items related to early breastfeeding management, explain how they might interfere with the mother's intentions relating to (a) breastfeeding initiation and (b) breastfeeding duration.

9. Review a week's discussions/archives of LACTNET or a similar email discussion group pertaining to breastfeeding. Describe the topics mentioned, and select two different points of view presented for two such topics. What do these discussions tell you about current concerns pertaining to lactation/breastfeeding?

10. Explain when you would use each of the following audiovisual aids in a presentation to (a) a class of pregnant couples and (b) a group of health care providers:
    a. slides
    b. transparencies
    c. videotape
    d. handouts

11. Select a brochure designed to inform mothers about some aspect of breastfeeding. Evaluate the brochure on the following elements:
    a. reading level
    b. compliance with WHO Code recommendations
    c. support of breastfeeding (general and specific)
    d. positive promotion of breastfeeding
    e. negative comments about breastfeeding
    f. suggestions supportive of nonbreastfeeding
    Provide examples of each of the elements above and defend your decision to use or not use the brochure in question.

Story Problem

You have been a staff member of a physicians' multispecialty clinic for five years. In response to increasing complaints from patients about the lack of consistent breastfeeding information and support, you are asked to present a plan designed to improve the clinic's reputation as a "breastfeeding-friendly" care setting.

1. Why might you initially refuse the job?

2. What do you finally present to the medical staff? (An outline will do.)

3. Select two elements from your outline, and add flesh to the bones of your proposal.

4. Explain where two forms of antagonism originate: one is overt; the other covert. Why have these reactions occurred, and how do you plan to counter them?

5. Who among the staff are enthusiastic about your proposal? Why?

After several months of discussion, but little action, you meet with a group of other staff members to plan a strategy of "deliberative change."

6. Who among the staff are members of this group? Why have you selected them – or have you?

7. Outline your strategy of "deliberative change."

8. Indicate the reasoning behind your selection of the order of elements you've incorporated into your plan for change.

9. How do you plan to evaluate the effectiveness of your step-by-step plan? When do you plan to do such an evaluation? Why?

10. Where does patient education fit into your plan? Why there, rather than earlier or later?

THE BREASTFEEDING PROCESS: THE PERINATAL AND INTRAPARTUM PERIOD

Outline

Key Concepts

You are urged to look for these key concepts in the body of the chapter and to develop questions deriving from these concepts as one way to gain understanding and insight into their relationship to lactation and breastfeeding. In this chapter, you are asked to evaluate policies and practices of a local birthing center against the breastfeeding management recommendations offered. Note where current care patterns are appropriate practice and where practices need to be changed or protocols developed in order to incorporate newer practices into care plans.

Blood sugar values

Breast fullness

Breast refusal

Cluster feedings

Discharge planning

Engorgement

Feeding plan

Feeding positions

Hand expression

Self care

Suckling pattern

Supplementation methods

Multiple-Choice Questions

1. Rubbing the nipples and areola with a towel has been suggested as a way of preparing the nipples for breastfeeding. How do you respond to a question about doing so?
   a. It is unnecessary and can make the mother more, rather than less, tender.
   b. It is appropriate if the mother is extremely gentle.
   c. It is appropriate if the mother succeeds in feeling a burning sensation; this means it is working.
   d. It is necessary only if the mother has very pale pink, or freckled, skin.

2. Following an unexpected cesarean birth, a mother
   a. should not attempt to breastfeed.
   b. will not need help from a visiting nurse.
   c. may feel that she has failed as a woman.
   d. will not make enough milk to nourish her baby fully.

3. When adjusting the infant for the first feedings using a cradle hold, the neonate should be positioned so that his body
   a. is rotated upward.
   b. faces away from his mother.
   c. faces the health care provider so that he can be observed.
   d. faces his mother.

4. Hoffman's exercises may
   a. evert a previously inverted nipple, according to recent research reports.
   b. prevent early nipple tenderness in the primiparous mother.
   c. help a mother become more matter-of-fact about handling her breasts.
   d. cause further retraction of a partially retracted nipple.

5. A problem of too much milk
   a. almost never occurs in the developed world.
   b. occurs only when the baby receives too much hindmilk.
   c. occurs only when the baby receives too much foremilk.
   d. is most likely when the baby breastfeeds frequently and effectively.

6. Studies have shown that, when baby-friendly concepts are incorporated into hospital care routines,
   a. more mothers are likely to breastfeed for a longer period.
   b. fewer mothers are likely to breastfeed for a longer period.
   c. more mothers are likely to breastfeed in the hospital, but not later.
   d. fewer mothers are likely to breastfeed in the hospital, but more after they are discharged.

7. Epidural anesthesia/analgesia
   a. has no known effects on the breastfeeding newborn.
   b. may delay the time to the baby's effective breastfeeding.
   c. may speed up the time to the baby's effective breastfeeding.
   d. usually affects breastfeeding only when it is given to primiparous mothers.

8. The BEST intervention for engorgement is
   a. avoiding breast pumping because it will stimulate milk production.
   b. applying warm cabbage leaves to the breasts.
   c. applying cool, moist towels to the breasts and pumping to relief.
   d. applying hot, dry towels to the breasts and pumping to relief.

9. In assisting the mother to put her infant to breast, wait for _____ before placing the infant on the breast.
   a. the widest point of the rooting reflex - the infant's gape
   b. the infant to start rooting
   c. the infant to begin suckling
   d. the infant to cry to signal a desire to feed

10. During hand expression, the mother presses _____ toward the chest wall, squeezing gently with a slight _____ action toward the chest wall.
    a. upward, rolling
    b. downward, rotating
    c. inward, rotating
    d. inward, rolling

Short-Answer Questions

1. Identify at least three different ways in which a mother can prepare for breastfeeding.

2. Identify and briefly discuss at least five different fallacies or faulty assumptions pertaining to breastfeeding. Note why these assumptions are faulty, and offer a more appropriate alternative explanation of the issue in question.

3. Identify three different ways of holding a baby for breastfeeding. In each case, specify when a mother might use each position and at least one caution pertaining to each.

4. What is hypoglycemia? Identify when it is most likely to occur in a neonate, and explain the rationale for how the baby should be managed.

5. Answer each of the following questions with a sentence or two that characterizes a normal suckling pattern in the healthy newborn:
   a. What do the baby's cheeks look like?
   b. Where is the baby's tongue?
   c. What do you hear when the baby is suckling?
   d. How tight is the baby's seal on the breast?

6. Briefly explain what colic is, noting at least three different explanations for its occurrence in some babies.

7. Explain why the best breastfeeding classes are taught by independent lactation consultants.

8. Briefly distinguish between typical stooling patterns in an exclusively breastfed baby and a baby receiving only artificial baby milk at the following time periods:
   a. day 2
   b. day 10
   c. day 30
   d. day 80

9. Briefly describe finger feeding, and why it might be used.

10. Explain the usual pattern of glucose levels in the newborn and when it is most appropriate to secure a blood glucose level.

11. Review the four patterns of breast engorgement identified by Humenick et al. Outline a study protocol that would enable you to determine how frequently each of these patterns occurs in a sample of 100 consecutive women giving birth at the same community hospital.

12. Describe the circumstances under which a thin silicone nipple shield might be used to assist breastfeeding. What cautions would you offer the mother?

Essay Questions

1. Discuss at least four different reasons why early and frequent breastfeeding promotes optimal functioning in both mother and newborn. Show how each reason is related to the other reasons you have selected.

2. Distinguish between breast fullness and breast engorgement, noting when each is likely to occur. Briefly indicate how you would characterize each so that a mother could tell when they occur and would know what to do for herself following discharge from the birthing center as soon as 12 hours after the birth.

3. You are approached by a sales representative who is eager for your endorsement of a new nipple and breast cream which is soon to be released to the market in all English-speaking countries. What is your reply to the sales representative? Justify your answer with three different reasons supporting your decision.

4. A mother comes to your office complaining that she thinks she doesn't have "enough milk" to feed her baby. Her baby is now 11 weeks old. The baby is in the 75th percentile for height and the 50th percentile for weight. Identify at least five factors relating to the baby and at least five other factors relating to the mother which may have contributed to the mother's conclusion that she hasn't enough milk. For each factor, offer her a one- or two-sentence explanation designed to answer her concerns.

5. What is discharge planning? Identify at least two areas of teaching that help the mother as she continues to breastfeed. Identify three signs that indicate the need for intervention.

6. Examine the Endresen and Helsing, and the Wright et al. studies. Using them as a model, outline a plan for incorporating BFHI concepts into a hospital's care routines. Which steps would you implement first, and why? Which steps would you expect to have the greatest impact on (a) breastfeeding initiation and (b) breastfeeding duration? What evidence would you gather to support your claims?

Story Problem

You, as a lactation consultant, have recently joined a group of physicians - including one obstetrician, two family practitioners (one of whom practices obstetrics), one pediatrician, and one internal medicine specialist. One of the physicians is less informed about breastfeeding than her partners. One of your roles is to provide prenatal breastfeeding instruction to all pregnant families.

1. Briefly outline the contents of your breastfeeding class, noting how you will respond to questions.

In addition to providing prenatal instruction, you are also expected to see all new mothers and babies during their hospital stay.

2. Describe what you do in the hospital with these clients. How do you reply when one of the nurses on the postpartum unit asks why you ask the mothers to sit up in a chair, rather than lounge back in the bed, for early breastfeedings?

One of the mothers you saw in the hospital is breastfeeding without difficulty. Her roommate is faring less well. Her baby rarely stays on the breast more than one minute before appearing to fall asleep. By day three, the mother is severely engorged; her baby is jaundiced and bili-lights have been ordered for use at home after her discharge this afternoon.

3. How do you assist this mother without increasing the other mother's anxiety? What do you tell the mother about reducing her engorgement and encouraging the baby to be more wakeful for feedings?

After the mother is discharged, you are unsuccessful in reaching her at home. A week later she calls you. Her baby is nursing better, and the engorgement is gone, but she was quite disappointed to learn from the doctor that her baby has not regained his birth weight. This particular physician feels that every full-term infant should have regained birth weight within seven days.

4. How do you respond to the mother's questions about having to use supplements without calling into question the doctor's comments to her?

THE BREASTFEEDING PROCESS: THE POSTPARTUM PERIOD

Outline

Adequate hydration and nutrition of the neonate

Insufficient milk supply (IMS)

Perceived Insufficient milk supply

Actual or primary insufficient milk supply

Breast massage

Sore nipples

Neonatal physiological jaundice

Crying and colic

Stooling patterns

Changes over time

Stooling as an indication of a problem

Multiple infants

Refusing the breast

Too much milk

Leaking and breast pads

Clothing

Breastfeeding during pregnancy

Clinical implications

Key Concepts

Breast massage

Breast refusal

Colic

Crying

Hydration

Insufficient milk supply

Leaking

Milk transfer

Multiple infants

Nipple tenderness

Stooling

Sucking patterns

Multiple-Choice Questions

1. According to the American Academy of Pediatrics, the new mother-infant dyad should be discharged when
   a. the mothers chooses to go home.
   b. the insurance company coverage has been exhausted.
   c. at least two feedings with documentation of coordinated suckling, swallowing, and breathing have occurred.
   d. the baby has been observed to feed on a bottle with coordinated suckling, swallowing, and breathing.

2. Insufficient milk supply
   a. is a problem that occurs in approximately 70 percent of babies of primiparous mothers.
   b. can be resolved most rapidly if the mother is asked to supplement the baby for the first two weeks of life.
   c. is almost never a problem in the developed world.
   d. is often perceived even in the absence of verification that the baby needs more milk.

3. The mother of multiples needs to
   a. accept that she will probably have to supplement at least one baby.
   b. accept the help of friends during the early weeks postpartum.
   c. remember that psychological attachment is more likely when one baby comes home before the other(s).
   d. sit up for all breastfeedings in order to nurse more than one baby at a time.

4. When a baby refuses to feed on one breast, but will go to the other,
   a. the baby may be indicating that he can see better out of one eye than the other.
   b. the mother will need to supplement the baby to assure that growth continues.
   c. the baby may be indicating that a benign cyst is present in the breast.
   d. the mother will be able to adequately nourish the baby.

5. What is milk transfer?
   a. movement of the milk bottles from the porch to the refrigerator
   b. movement of the milk from the mother's breasts into the baby's mouth
   c. movement of the milk from the baby's mouth into his intestines
   d. movement of milk that is painful to the mother - as when a cyst is present

6. Breast massage should be practiced
    a. just before or while the baby is feeding, to enhance letdown.
    b. only when the baby is off the breast.
    c. only when the mother has cysts that prevent the free flow of milk.
    d. only when the mother has breast cancer, to prevent the baby from getting cancer cells.

7. When would transitory nipple soreness be most noticeable?
    a. between the first and second postpartum day
    b. between the third and sixth postpartum day
    c. between the sixth and tenth postpartum day
    d. any time in the first two weeks, depending on the mother's complexion

8. The top priority discharge teaching for breastfeeding families is
    a. normal stooling and wetting patterns of neonates.
    b. the best type of clothing to wear for discreet breastfeeding.
    c. where the mother can obtain a breast pump.
    d. coping with a crying baby.

9. The neonate should be expected to regain his birth weight no later than ___ postpartum.
    a. five days
    b. one week
    c. two weeks
    d. three weeks

10. Based on research outcomes, these two treatments appear to alleviate sore nipples:
    a. purified lanolin and Massé cream
    b. purified lanolin and warm water
    c. aloe vera and warm water
    d. chapstick and vitamin E oil

11. Crying is a _____ indicator of the need to feed.
    a. first
    b. very early
    c. intermediate
    d. late

Short-Answer Questions

1. Provide the rationale for using 7 percent weight loss as a marker for additional evaluation, and 10 percent weight loss as a red flag of problems occurring in the breastfeeding dyad.

2. Identify and discuss at least three cues the mother might conclude are evidence that she does not have enough milk. How would you inform the mother that those cues mean something else? What might they mean?

3. What is a cluster feeding, and how might the mother identify it?

4. What is the relationship between postpartum hemorrhage and later breastfeeding difficulty?

5. Discuss at least three different factors that appear to be related to colic. How might each such explanation be discussed with the mother so that she sees that breastfeeding need not be interrupted or stopped completely?

6. Describe the breastfeeding baby's usual stool pattern, distinguishing between the first week, the first month, and later times. What particular differences do you feel should be emphasized when working with a new mother?

Essay Questions

1. Distinguish between transient sore nipples and prolonged, abnormal sore nipples. What might cause each type? How might each of these problems be resolved?

2. Describe two different factors that can contribute to breast refusal. How would you help the mother solve this problem for each factor contributing to the problem?

3. What is overactive letdown reflex? How would you identify it? What would you suggest to the mother to resolve this difficulty?

Story Problem

You are the LC at Community Hospital. You've just said good-bye to a new mother, Adelle who gave birth to Adam 40 hours ago.

1. What three items did you emphasize in the discharge planning you had with her a few minutes ago? Why did you focus her attention on those three items?

2. Adelle calls you in tears. The baby didn't sleep all last night and now is refusing to breastfeed. What do you tell her?

3. Adelle calls you back. Your suggestions haven't worked. The baby still won't take the breast. You decide to do a home visit.
   What do you observe upon entering the house? (mention presence/absence of relatives, friends)

The baby is now mouthing the nipple, but not really latching on well. What factors that occurred in the hospital may be contributing to this baby's behavior? What do you suggest now?

4. Four hours after your visit, Adelle leaves a message on your answering machine. "My mother says I should use a nipple shield. She brought one with her. What do you think?"
   What questions do you ask her about the nipple shield? What do you then tell her?

5. You aren't covered for more than one home visit, and you feel that Adelle needs additional help. Who, in the community, do you call? What do you tell Adelle? Her doctor is not convinced that breastfeeding mothers need help. "After all, isn't breastfeeding instinctive?"

6. Two days later, Adelle calls you. She is ecstatic. "It worked!" she fairly shouts into the phone. "What worked?" you ask. (So? Tell us what worked!)

11

SLOW WEIGHT GAIN AND FAILURE TO THRIVE

Outline

Key Concepts

You are urged to look for these key concepts in the body of the chapter and to develop questions deriving from these concepts as one way to gain understanding and insight into their relationship to lactation and breastfeeding. Pay attention to the similarities and differences between a healthy, slow-gaining infant and one who is failing to thrive. Noting important cues in a careful history and observing a breastfeeding encounter help determine the diagnosis and how best to support an optimal breastfeeding course.

Disorganized suckling

Failure to thrive

Growth charts

Hypothyroidism

Inadequate caloric intake

Insufficient feedings

Insufficient glandular tissue

Neurologic dysfunction

Normal growth

Positioning

Slow-gaining

Supplementation devices

Tongue-tie

Multiple-Choice Questions

1. Which of the following drugs has been used to build up a low maternal milk supply?
   a. metoclopramide
   b. chlorindione
   c. ciprofloxacin
   d. chloramphenicol

2. A baby with a disorganized suckle
   a. is usually older than one month of age.
   b. requires careful digital training to learn how to strip the lactiferous sinuses.
   c. may have been born prematurely.
   d. is often a twin.

3. Insufficient glandular tissue is a problem
   a. for approximately 50 percent of women in the developed world.
   b. that explains nearly all infant failure to thrive.
   c. that is relatively rare.
   d. that is secondary to the use of antihistamines.

4. Approximately what percentage of infants have been found to be gaining weight poorly as a result of an underlying organic problem?
   a. 85 percent
   b. 60 percent
   c. 40 percent
   d. 20 percent

5. Which of the following growth parameters is most likely to suggest early failure to thrive?
   a. infant weight
   b. infant head circumstance
   c. length/height
   d. chest circumference

6. About how much should a baby gain in length by his first year anniversary?
   a. approximately 25 percent of his length at birth
   b. approximately double his length at birth
   c. approximately 10 percent of his length at birth
   d. approximately 50 percent of his length at birth

7. The baby is expected to gain approximately 3 inches in head circumference in his first year of life. How does this relate to later increases in head circumference?
   a. He will gain another 3 inches in the next 3 years of life.
   b. He will gain another 3 inches in the next 16 years of life.
   c. He will gain another inch for every 3 years of additional life to age 16.
   d. He will gain another 2 inches for every 5 years of additional life to age 16.

8. All things being equal,
   a. milk production is related more to effective breastfeeding by the baby than to maternal ability to make milk.
   b. milk production is related more to maternal ability to make milk than to effective breastfeeding by the baby.
   c. milk production is related more to maternal nutritional status than to size of the baby at birth.
   d. milk production is related more to size of the baby at birth than to maternal nutritional status.

9. Both breastfed and formula-fed infants gain about _____ per day at one month of age.
   a. one-half ounce
   b. one ounce
   c. two ounces
   d. three ounces

10. Immediate care for a baby who is failing to thrive includes all EXCEPT
    a. monitoring fluid intake and output.
    b. testing the baby's developmental level.
    c. referral to a physician, preferably a pediatrician.
    d. supplementation: feed the baby.

Short-Answer Questions

1. What is tongue-tie? How do you identify it?

2. Please explain the relationship of each of the following to inadequate infant weight gain and what you would recommend to clients:
   a. suboptimal positioning
   b. insufficient numbers of feedings
   c. limited feeding length
   d. maternal hypothyroidism
   e. oral contraceptives and sedatives

3. Distinguish between infants with transitory and long-lasting neurological difficulties and how each might affect the breastfeeding course.

4. Briefly explain why detecting swallowing is important when attempting to determine the causes of infant failure to thrive.

5. What is the relationship between infant weight gain and maternal milk production? Offer two examples, one that suggests the baby's suckling prompted inadequate milk production and one that suggests the mother's milk production was inadequate to sustain appropriate infant growth.

6. As a rule of thumb, what are two indicators of poor weight gain in a breastfeeding baby?

7. Briefly explain the role of genetic tendencies in patterns of infant weight gain. Please provide two different examples to support your answer.

8. Briefly define how one would conclude that a baby is gaining weight slowly but is not failing to thrive.

9. How is infant fatness related to cream content of the mother's milk? What evidence supports your claim?

10. Explain why the growth rate seen in artificially fed babies in the first year of life can be considered to be excessive.

11. Compare how breastfed and artificially fed infants feed following the introduction of solid foods. How might these differences affect growth rate thereafter?

12. What is growth faltering, and how might it best be identified in a group of infants living in a developed country? a developing country?

13. How might the mother's own dietary restriction regimen be related to her infant's rate of gain?

14. Explain how establishing a 3 to 3.5-hour schedule of feedings in the first month of life might contribute to infant failure to thrive.

15. What is the relationship between pacifier (dummy) use, nipple preference/confusion, and subsequent failure to thrive?

16. How would you distinguish between a satiated baby, a sleepy baby, and a baby who is suffering failure to thrive when all have their eyes closed while at the breast?

Essay Questions

1. Identify at least four conditions that can result in infant failure to thrive. In each case identify how the condition might be identified, and develop a plan of care for the breastfeeding mother.

2. What is a "flutter suck" and how does it relate to poor weight gain in the baby?

3. Explain how growth charts were devised and why they are sometimes considered problematic when evaluating growth patterns in breastfed infants.

4. Briefly describe what is considered a "normal" pattern of growth in a human infant, paying attention to three different indices of growth.

5. Using one representative of each of the infants described by Butte and colleagues, explain how
   a. missed nighttime feedings may or may not increase the likelihood of FTT.
   b. milk intake might not differ in these two groups of infants.
   c. how you might use this information to
      (1)   encourage more frequent feedings for a baby whose rate of gain is slow.
      (2)   encourage more frequent feedings for a baby who has ceased gaining weight.
      (3)   reassure a mother who is concerned about her baby's growth, which is found to be within the 50th percentile for length and age.

Story Problem

A client with a five-week-old infant is referred for evaluation of inadequate infant weight gain. The referring physician's note includes the following information:

> *Baby boy Jones was born following an uneventful pregnancy to a 28-year-old primipara who claims to be breastfeeding "on demand." Birth weight was 6 lbs., 14 oz.; weight at four weeks was 6 lbs., 2 oz. Length at birth was 19"; length at four weeks was 19-1/2". Maternal behavior is inconsistent with infant neglect. Evaluation for organic disease is negative.*

1. Based on the above information, what do you suspect?

During your first appointment with the mother you take a history.

2. Based on that history, identify at least two different management issues that may have contributed to this baby's pattern of weight loss. Indicate how you've identified these issues and what intervention(s) you might recommend to overcome them.

3. Identify two additional maternal factors that may be implicated in this situation. Indicate how you've identified these factors and what interventions you recommend to overcome them.

4. Identify two other infant factors that may be contributing to the baby's poor weight gain. Indicate how you've identified these factors and what interventions you recommend to overcome them.

After taking the history, you ask the mother to breastfeed. Her baby has remained alert and quiet, with occasional fussing, but was quieted by use of a pacifier during the 90 minutes of history taking and discussion.

5. Describe <u>how</u> the mother brings her baby to the breast.

6. Describe <u>how</u> the infant suckles.

7. After observing the mother and baby breastfeeding, you suspect you know why the baby is gaining weight poorly. Explain what you observed that suggests an explanation.

8. Tell us what you then say to the mother to help her understand why her baby is gaining weight poorly.

9. Now indicate why you rule out a diagnosis of normal slow weight gain and conclude that the baby is failing to thrive.

You offer the mother several suggestions about how to get extra milk into the baby.

10. How does she respond to each of the following alternatives?
    a. a bottle after every breastfeeding
    b. cup-feeding after every breastfeeding
    c. spoon-feeding after every breastfeeding
    d. pumping her breasts
    e. breastfeeding the baby at least once (more) at night than has been occurring
    f. using a feeding tube device

11. About how much milk per feeding do you suggest that the mother put in the feeding tube device or other container she is using to give the baby extra fluid?

12. How do you answer the mother when she insists on knowing when she can "go back to just breastfeeding whenever my baby wants to"?

12

JAUNDICE AND THE BREASTFEEDING BABY

Outline

Early-onset (neonatal) jaundice

Pathological jaundice

Factors associated with early-onset jaundice

    Infant characteristics

    Hospital routines

Routine therapy for early-onset jaundice

Incipient vulnerable child syndrome: One cost of overdiagnosis

Late-onset jaundice

Clinical implications

Key Concepts

You are urged to look for these key concepts in the body of the chapter and to develop questions deriving from these concepts as one way to gain understanding and insight into their relationship to lactation and breastfeeding. In this chapter, you may find it helpful to consider how jaundice in the neonatal period is viewed in your community and compare it to the presentation in this chapter. Where differences exist, one useful exercise would be to identify these differences and note when differences between current practice and suggested recommendations from this chapter can be reconciled with minimum disruption.

Conjugated bilirubin

Early-onset jaundice

Incipient vulnerable child syndrome

Late-onset jaundice

Nonhuman milk feeds

Pathologic jaundice

Serum bilirubin

"Starvation-induced" jaundice

Unconjugated bilirubin

Water supplementation

Multiple-Choice Questions

1. Which of the following characterizes late-onset jaundice?
   a. It is present in 70 percent to 100 percent of all breastfed infants.
   b. In most cases it requires no intervention.
   c. In most cases it requires interruption of breastfeeding.
   d. It often occurs within the first five days postbirth.

2. Which of the following characterizes early-onset jaundice?
   a. It usually manifests itself within 24 hours after birth.
   b. In most cases it requires a 24-hour interruption of breastfeeding.
   c. It is more likely when the baby feeds infrequently.
   d. It is more likely when the baby receives additional milk feedings.

3. Which of the following reduces serum bilirubin levels in neonates?
   a. short, frequent feedings of glucose water
   b. frequent, unlimited breastfeedings
   c. breastfeeding approximately every three to four hours with supplements of glucose water between feeds as needed
   d. bililight therapy from day two through day four

4. "Starvation-induced" jaundice can occur when babies are
   a. fed frequently at the breast.
   b. given water or glucose in place of milk feedings.
   c. fed nonhuman milk.
   d. breastfed exclusively.

5. Fetal hemoglobin
   a. picks up oxygen poorly.
   b. has a high affinity for oxygen.
   c. enables the baby to grow rapidly in a highly oxygenated environment.
   d. enhances lung breathing after birth.

6. Jaundice in the three-day-old term neonate reflects
   a. increased concentrations of fat-soluble bilirubin.
   b. increased concentrations of water-soluble bilirubin.
   c. decreased concentrations of fat-soluble bilirubin.
   d. increasing amounts of protein in human milk.

7. Kernicterus
   a. is unheard of and unproved to exist in breastfed infants.
   b. can occur when bilirubin levels exceed 30 mg/dL.
   c. can occur when bilirubin levels exceed 15 mg/dL.
   d. is more likely if the baby receives milk feedings but no water feedings.

8. Which of the following ethnic/racial groups have the highest bilirubin levels on day three?
   a. Asian or Indian neonates
   b. Hispanic neonates
   c. Caucasian neonates
   d. African neonates

9. Which of the following neonates is LEAST likely to become jaundiced?
   a. lighter- rather than heavier-weight healthy term infants
   b. infants born to mothers with diabetes
   c. preterm infants
   d. term infants

10. When a baby is diagnosed as jaundiced, how can this affect the mother's perception of her newborn?
    a. She may perceive him or her to have a life-threatening condition.
    b. She may perceive him or her to be protected from a life-threatening condition.
    c. She may perceive him or her to need less illness or wellness care.
    d. There appears to be no relationship between maternal perceptions and a diagnosis of jaundice in the neonate.

Short-Answer Questions

1. Briefly describe the rationale behind each of the following questions as it relates to minimizing the likelihood of early-onset jaundice.
   a. How often is the infant put to breast?
   b. How is the baby suckling?
   c. What is the baby's stooling pattern?
   d. Besides breastmilk, what other fluids is the baby being given?
   e. When is the baby being breastfed during any 24-hour period?

2. Briefly explain why Asian babies have higher serum bilirubin levels than Caucasian or black babies. What implications does this finding have for care relating to early-onset jaundice in Asian babies?

3. A mother is asked to stop breastfeeding for two days in order for her jaundiced three-day old baby to receive milk other than her own. The rationale for this request is not made clear to her. What would you tell her so that she understands the reasoning behind this request? Indicate why you consider this request appropriate or inappropriate in the overall care plan established for her baby.

4. Briefly describe "incipient vulnerable child syndrome" and how a diagnosis of jaundice may contribute to it.

5. What is pathological jaundice? When is it likely to manifest itself?

6. Describe body-wrap phototherapy. Identify potential benefits and risks of this kind of bilirubin therapy.

7. Explain why late-onset jaundice is often a diagnosis of exclusion.

8. Explain how heat treatment of human milk can reduce the likelihood of continued elevation in the recipient infant's hyperbilirubinemia.

9. Explain why the bottle-fed neonate could be described as overfed in the first three days of life and how this might influence bilirubin levels in such a neonate.

Essay Questions

1. Care of the jaundiced neonate often includes routines that have recently been questioned. Identify at least four such hospital routines, and note at least two effects of those routines on the neonate that could contribute to an elevation in bilirubin. Also note whether and/or how these same routines could contribute to difficulty with breastfeeding.

2. The authors of this chapter state: "It is appropriate to examine those routines which can be most easily altered or eliminated to reduce the likelihood that initiation of infant feeding *of any kind* in that institution contributes to early-onset jaundice." What do they mean by this statement?

3. Briefly distinguish between early-onset jaundice and late-onset jaundice, noting at least four differences between them.

4. Select at least four variables that have been found to influence the likelihood of the occurrence of "breastfeeding jaundice." Explain the significance of each of these variables to one another and to the likelihood of bilirubin elevation.

5. Discuss the pros and cons of each of the following treatment options when the newborn has a serum bilirubin >17 mg/dL.
   a. continue breastfeeding and observe
   b. interrupt breastfeeding and feed formula
   c. interrupt breastfeeding, feed formula, and begin phototherapy
   d. continue breastfeeding and begin phototherapy

6. Describe how each of the following characteristics of infants can influence the likelihood of occurrence of early-onset jaundice:
   a. racial/ethnic group
   b. birth weight
   c. stool patterns
   d. weight loss

7. Discuss the following hospital routines and how they may increase or decrease the likelihood of severity of hyperbilirubinemia:
   a. analgesia/anesthesia
   b. type of feeding
   c. frequency of feeding
   d. supplemental milk feedings
   e. supplemental water feedings

Story Problem

You receive a phone call from Monica Tremain. Her first baby was considered to be severely jaundiced (serum bilirubin levels on day two were 15 and on day three were 18) and required bililight therapy for several days before coming home. As a result, Monica stopped breastfeeding; she was convinced that her milk was the reason for the baby's yellow skin and lethargy. This mother is due to give birth to her second child in two weeks. She would like to breastfeed this baby, but she is fearful that her milk is "bad."

1. What do you ask her about her experience with her first baby?

2. What do you tell her to expect with this new baby?

Monica gives birth to a healthy boy, who shows an immediate interest in suckling for extended periods. After seeing colostrum dribble out of the baby's mouth, Monica exclaims, "Look how yellow that is! No wonder Gisele was so yellow!"

3. What is your response?

Gunter continues to suckle well throughout the hospital stay. On day three, the pediatrician reports to Monica that the baby's bilirubin level is 9. The doctor would prefer that it be lower and asks Monica to bring the baby in the next day for another blood sample. In the meantime, she is to supplement the baby with water after every feeding to "flush" the baby's system.

4. How do you respond when Monica – convinced that her milk has again done something to her baby – tearfully relates this conversation to you? If your recommendation differs from the doctor's, how do you reconcile the two so that Monica continues to view her doctor as supportive of breastfeeding?

The next day, Monica learns that the baby's serum bilirubin has dropped to 3. She calls you triumphant; but she continues to harbor concerns because "the doctor told me it's now too low!"

5. What do you tell Monica this time?

BREAST PUMPS AND OTHER TECHNOLOGIES

Outline

Breast shells

    Recommendations on breast shells

Feeding-tube devices

    Description

    Situations for use

Clinical implications

Key Concepts

You are urged to look for these key concepts in the body of the chapter and to develop questions deriving from these concepts as one way to gain understanding and insight into their relationship to lactation and breastfeeding. In this chapter, you may find it helpful to identify the array of breastfeeding technologies available to mothers in your community. Noting the problems these technologies have represented may help you to use the information in the chapter to assess whether the technologies are appropriate or inappropriate and make recommendations that reduce the difficulties in using such devices.

Breast pumps

Breast shells

Feeding-tube devices

Finger feeding

Milk-ejection reflex

Nipple shields

Multiple-Choice Questions

1. For optimal response to a breast pump, the milk-ejection reflex should be elicited
   a. before the mother begins pumping her breast.
   b. at the time the mother begins pumping her breast.
   c. after the mother has been pumping her breast at least two minutes.
   d. as long as milk begins to flow during the pumping session; when the milk-ejection reflex occurs is immaterial.

2. Which of the following devices is most often a source of milk contamination?
   a. intermittent electric pumps
   b. breast shells
   c. feeding-tube devices
   d. battery-operated breast pumps

3. Which of the following instructions relates to the use of nipple shields?
   a. Ask the mother to sign a consent form identifying the risks of using the device.
   b. Suggest that, once it is begun, it needs to continue to be used until the baby weans.
   c. Suggest that only neurologically impaired babies benefit from its use.
   d. Suggest that premature babies are too immature to use a nipple shield well.

4. Nearly all of the breastfeeding devices in existence today
   a. are the products of a high-tech society.
   b. reflect a societal predisposition to think of breastfeeding as difficult.
   c. reflect earlier versions of devices invented hundreds of years ago.
   d. signify the breastfeeding mother's need for assistance.

5. When a mother uses a breast pump, she is likely to obtain the most milk
   a. in the evening.
   b. in the morning.
   c. immediately after the baby has breastfed.
   d. whenever she has waited at least three hours since the last pumping session.

6. Maternal milk storage capacity is a function of
   a. the mother's parity.
   b. the baby's age.
   c. the breast size.
   d. the timing of breast pumping sessions.

7. The milk-ejection reflex produces
   a. a decrease in intramammary pressure.
   b. a later increase in oxytocin secretion.
   c. a later increase in prolactin secretion.
   d. an increase in intramammary pressure.

8. A mother has difficulty getting her baby to latch. What piece of equipment might she be tempted to use to solve this problem?
   a. a breast pump
   b. a breast shell
   c. a nipple shield
   d. a feeding-tube device

9. In order for a baby to use a feeding tube device, the baby
   a. should be able to latch and suckle.
   b. need not be able to latch.
   c. should not be jaundiced.
   d. should be at least 39 weeks' gestational age.

Short-Answer Questions

1. Identify at least two alternatives to using a nipple shield. Explain why you would recommend each alternative.

2. What is the significance of the amount of pressure that can be generated by different breast pumps? What would you caution mothers regarding the generation of maximum pressure? maintaining adequate pressure?

3. What is finger feeding? When is it an appropriate alternative to bottle-feeding? Identify a major risk involving its use.

4. Briefly explain why nipple shields are sometimes referred to as a "quick-fix" approach to early breastfeeding problems. How is this approach related to their inappropriate use?

5. Briefly distinguish between different types of breast shells, noting at least one risk and benefit of each.

6. Identify two different problems women sometimes encounter when they use breast pumps. Briefly explain how you would assist a mother in overcoming these problems.

7. Briefly explain why there is no such thing as one pump that works for all women.

8. Describe the four phases of a breast pumping cycle. Explain how each is related to infant suckling.

9. What is backflow, and how can it be avoided?

10. Obtain pricing information for at least four different breast pumps available in your area. Note (1) initial cost to purchase; (2) rental price per day, week, month, or longer and (3) availability of replacement parts. Based on this information, which pump appears to be the most cost-effective for
    a. a mother planning to pump occasionally.
    b. a mother who is returning to work within six weeks of her baby's birth.
    c. a mother whose 27-week gestational age preterm baby is in a hospital 100 miles away.
    d. a mother who must be hospitalized for gall bladder surgery.

11. Review the instructions accompanying two different breast pumps or kits. Identify
    a. information that is accurate.
    b. information that is confusing.
    c. information that may not accurately reflect the lactation process.
    In each case, how will such information affect user satisfaction with the device in question?

12. Describe finger feeding and at least two situations when it might be used.

Essay Questions

1. Identify all of the different breastfeeding-related technologies available in your community. With which of these items have you had personal experience? experience through a client's use of one or more of them? What problems have the devices been used to solve? What problems have the devices themselves posed?

2. Identify at least six different uses for a feeding-tube device: three involving maternal situations and three involving infant situations. In each case, indicate how the feeding-tube device can assist in feeding or resolve the problem presented.

3. Identify at least three problems that can occur with the use of breast shells. Distinguish between their use prenatally and in the postpartum period.

4. Identify six different characteristics of a breast pump, noting for each characteristic its importance for the breastfeeding mother.

5. Outline a proposed study to examine the efficacy of four different models of breast pumps such that their performance can be compared. Identify in your proposal how you would avoid the following problems:
   a. retrospective recall failure of users
   b. inappropriate comparisons
   c. measurement errors pertaining to milk volume obtained
   d. user preferences for certain pumps

Story Problem

Marie has called your office to ask for a consultation in advance of her baby's birth. She is interested in obtaining a breast pump, which she plans to use after delivery.

1. What information do you need to know before recommending a pump?

2. Under what circumstances would you recommend *against* using a breast pump?

Marie leaves your office without a pump; she has chosen to wait until after the baby is born before obtaining one. You see her a week later and learn that one nipple inverts with pressure, while the other one is everted. The baby prefers the everted one.

3. How do you help Marie?

4. Which device will you use, if any, to assist the baby in learning to take Marie's inverted nipple?

Marie's husband is skeptical about the use of any breastfeeding devices; he prefers to think of lactation as "natural."

5. How do you support his view while assisting Marie as she uses one or more devices?

6. Which devices has she chosen to use?

When Marie next has contact with you, it is because she thinks the baby has thrush. After seeing both of them, you concur with her.

7. Why do you recommend that she use a breast shell during the period when her baby and her breasts are being treated?

A week later, a mother with a baby whose suck is extremely weak is referred to you by a physician.

8. How do you recommend that the mother get adequate amounts of milk into the baby?

9. What kind of milk do you recommend? Why?

10. If the mother is uncomfortable using a breast pump to increase her own supply, what do you recommend that she do?

11. What do you tell the baby's primary caregiver about your plans for this mother and baby?

This mother asks you how long you think it will take for her one-month-old baby to learn how to breast-feed correctly.

12. What is your reply? Explain the rationale behind your answer.

14

BREASTFEEDING THE PRETERM INFANT

Outline

Test weighing

Facilitating milk transfer

Milk ejection

Infant suckling

Breastfeeding devices

Postdischarge breastfeeding management

Getting enough: Milk-transfer problems

Practice implications

Key Concepts

You are urged to look for these key concepts in the body of the chapter and to develop questions deriving from these concepts as one way to gain understanding and insight into their relationship to lactation and breastfeeding. In this chapter, you may find it helpful to discuss whether certain issues that are important when the infant is premature are also important when the infant is a healthy, full-term neonate. In some cases, insight can also be gained by comparing the period of hospitalization with the postdischarge breastfeeding period.

Bacteriologic surveillance

Breastfeeding management

Expressed mothers' milk

Expression schedule

Feedings from different containers

Gavage feeding

Hindmilk feeding

Human milk fortification/modification

Milk transfer

Nonnutritive sucking

Skin-to-skin care

Test weighings

Multiple-Choice Questions

1. When a mother's infant is admitted to the NICU, she is considered a breastfeeding "candidate"
   a. when she says she wants to breastfeed.
   b. when she says she had planned to breastfeed.
   c. when the baby is able to suckle the breast.
   d. unless she indicates otherwise.

2. Indecisive mothers will often choose to breastfeed a preterm infant because
   a. they really do want to breastfeed.
   b. they recognize the health benefits of human milk for their baby.
   c. they are trying to make up for the pregnancy that ended too soon.
   d. they are told they must do so by the baby's physician.

3. In most cases, the mother of a preterm infant will find _____ most effective in obtaining milk.
   a. hand expression
   b. a hand-operated breast pump
   c. an electric breast pump
   d. a battery-operated breast pump

4. The composition of human milk is such that it meets
   a. none of the nutritional needs of the very low-birth-weight infant.
   b. only the nutritional needs of the term infant.
   c. the nutritional needs of the infant, regardless of his prematurity.
   d. some of the nutritional needs of the low-birth-weight infants.

5. Which of the following elements in human milk is NOT present in higher concentrations in the milk of a mother of a premature infant?
   a. short-chain fatty acids
   b. iron
   c. protein
   d. sIgA

6. Which of the following experiences is considered an inhibitor of prolactin secretion?
   a. the infant's health status
   b. a cesarean birth
   c. irregular breast emptying
   d. delay in getting the baby to breast

7. When advising a mother about the frequency of breast pumping following a premature birth, optimal recommendations include
   a. pumping up to four to six times a day.
   b. pumping for approximately 50 minutes in 24 hours.
   c. pumping for approximately 75 minutes in 24 hours.
   d. pumping eight to ten times a day.

8. When nonnutritive sucking occurs at breast, how does this affect the mother's milk supply?
   a. It takes away from the milk she is able to obtain with breast pumping.
   b. It may increase her milk production (volume obtained).
   c. It may cause confusion in the baby, who has previously used a pacifier for nonnutritive sucking.
   d. It may result in increased frustration in the mother, who expects the baby to get a full feeding from such exposure to the breast.

9. A preterm baby should be put to breast after he
   a. has maintained a weight of at least 1200 gms for three days.
   b. has shown that he can feed from a bottle without aspirating.
   c. has shown the ability to coordinate sucking and swallowing.
   d. no longer needs human milk fortifier.

Short-Answer Questions

1. Why should a milk expression schedule for the mother of a preterm infant parallel the frequency with which a healthy, full-term newborn breastfeeds?

2. What protocols ensure that expressed breastmilk for the preterm infant has minimal concentrations of bacteria?

3. Under what circumstances should a double-pumping collection kit be considered the standard of care?

4. Discuss each of the following barriers to in-hospital breastfeeding of the preterm infant:
   a. not providing an adequate environment in which to breastfeed the infant
   b. requiring that the baby reach a certain weight or age before being allowed to breastfeed
   c. requiring that the baby bottle-feed successfully before being given an opportunity to breastfeed

5. Briefly explain why routine test weighing is considered the standard of care for small preterm infants.

6. Briefly discuss the following elements as indicators of readiness to breastfeed:
   a. coordination of suck-swallow-breathing
   b. gestational age
   c. infant weight
   d. apneic episodes during bottle-feeding and during sleep

7. Explain why each of the following infant responses should be monitored and the results documented during early breastfeeding sessions. In each case, identify how they can be monitored, and indicate whether these are invasive or noninvasive.
   a. heart rate
   b. respiratory rate
   c. oxygen saturation or transcutaneous oxygen pressure ($TCPO_2$)
   d. body temperature
   e. test weighing

8. What is cue-based feeding? Give two examples of different cues that can be used when evaluating the preterm infant who has been breastfeeding for some time and has not yet been discharged from the hospital.

9. Briefly explain how you might answer a mother's questions about the appropriateness of continuing bottle-feedings after the baby has been discharged from the hospital.

10. Review what differences from term milk characterize the milk of mothers who have given birth prematurely. Why are these differences important for the premature infant?

11. Describe how to obtain an appropriate breast pump for a mother with limited financial resources following the birth of her premature baby.

12. Explain how one might provide hindmilk feedings and why this can help the preterm infant to grow.

13. What is skin-to-skin care, and how does it help the preterm infant?

Essay Questions

1. Identify and briefly describe three elements that should be included in an initial consultation with the mother of a preterm infant.

2. Identify at least three factors that are barriers to frequent milk expression. Discuss how each barrier can be overcome when developing an action plan with the mother of a preterm infant.

3. Briefly describe how expressed mothers' milk should be stored for later use.

4. The authors of this chapter note that there is an inverse relationship between infusion rate and lipid loss during gavage feedings. Why is this finding important? How might the effects of such a finding be minimized when caring for a preterm infant?

5. Briefly describe and demonstrate two different optimal positions for breastfeeding the premature infant. Explain when each position might be used.

6. Describe how the mother of a preterm infant newly admitted to the NICU ideally should be approached about providing her milk for her baby in a way that encourages her to consider breastfeeding.

7. Explain the rationale for preferring intermittent rather than slow-infusion continuous gavage feedings for preterm infants.

8. Review the pros and cons of mixing commercial milk fortifiers with a mother's own milk. What would you then advise a mother who asks you why her milk "is not good enough" for her baby?

9. Review the five principles offered in this chapter related to maternal medication use when the mother is providing milk for her preterm infant. Using these principles, develop guidelines that could be used in an NICU.

10. Describe how to assess milk transfer in the preterm infant and what you would instruct a mother to do so that she is reassured that such milk transfer is occurring, and that the baby is "getting enough."

Story Problem

Georgia Townsend has just arrived on the postpartum floor. Her twin sons were born by emergency cesarean section at 28 weeks gestational age. Georgia saw both babies only briefly before they were whisked away to the NICU. You are the lactation consultant who works with mothers whose babies are in the NICU.

1. Describe your first conversation with Georgia.

Georgia's roommate, Dorene, has a healthy baby whose cry is lusty and frequent. Dorene is bottle-feeding her baby. When you see Georgia on her first wheelchair visit to the NICU, she tells you she isn't sure she should breastfeed her babies, now named John, Jr., and Gilbert.

2. What is your response?

Georgia's husband, John, interrupts your conversation by insisting on showing her a piece of paper on which he has scribbled notes about what the doctor told him about their sons. One baby is on a respirator; the other needed such assistance for only the first 24 hours. He tells his wife that she <u>must</u> breastfeed because the doctor said the babies needed the milk. He looks to you for confirmation.

3. What is your response to his implied question?

Three days after Georgia gives birth, her first baby dies. You learn about this in a tearful phone call late at night. She hasn't pumped her breasts since learning of the baby's death six hours earlier. She says she feels "flat."

4. What do you suggest that she do between the time of the call and your first opportunity to see her later that day?

Georgia tells you that she still wants to give her milk to Gilbert. She asks if she will ever produce more than the 30cc that she is currently obtaining with the battery-operated breast pump she is using at home.

5. What is your response?

Four weeks later, when Gilbert is 32 weeks adjusted gestational age, the doctor considers him stable and ready to try to breastfeed. Georgia has been looking forward to this day; now that it has arrived she holds back. Her eyes filling with tears, she asks, "What if he doesn't like me?"

6. Now what do you do? Your reaction to the question, please.

To everyone's surprise and his mother's delight, little Gillie latches on to Georgia's left breast and suckles as if he has always been fed in this manner. He continues to suckle and swallow rhythmically in bursts, with longer pauses gradually predominating over 20 minutes. Then he falls into deep sleep.

7. What do you tell the baby's NICU nurse after this first breastfeeding?

8. What feeding plan do you then develop with Georgia and Gillie's primary nurse?

Three weeks after his first breastfeeding, Gilbert Townsend is discharged home. The pediatrician has asked Georgia and John to bring him to the office for a first visit in three days.

9. What do you tell Georgia about
    a. using the electric breast pump that she has been renting?
    b. breastfeeding Gillie?
    c. John's questions about "making sure" the baby gets enough milk by giving him two extra bottles a day?
    d. signs that Gillie doesn't need anything but the breast?
    e. her fears that she will "do something wrong"?
    f. who will be available to answer her questions and hold her hand?

BREAST-RELATED PROBLEMS

Outline

Key Concepts

You are urged to look for these key concepts in the body of the chapter and to develop questions deriving from these concepts as one way to gain understanding and insight into their relationship to lactation and breastfeeding. In this chapter, you are asked to consider how a variety of breast-related problems may influence the lactation course for the mother and her breastfeeding baby. Some of these problems will occur with relatively high frequency; others are considerably less likely. In all cases, however, the health of the mother and baby must be foremost when making recommendations.

Breast augmentation

Breast cancer

Breast reduction

Candidiasis

Fibrocystic breast disease

Intraductal papilloma

Inverted nipples

Mastitis

Mastopexy

Nursing diagnosis

Plugged duct

Prolactinomas

Multiple-Choice Questions

1. Which of the following is <u>MOST</u> likely to be associated with mastitis?
   a. plugged duct
   b. cracked nipple
   c. fatigue
   d. stasis

2. Prolactinomas
   a. are pituitary tumors.
   b. are a contraindication to breastfeeding.
   c. tend to grow wildly during lactation.
   d. are very likely to metastasize during lactation.

3. Women with a history of treatment for breast cancer
   a. should not consider breastfeeding.
   b. are unable to breastfeed after the surgery and/or chemotherapy.
   c. represent many unanswered questions for the medical community.
   d. are rarely able to produce milk with sufficient fats for the baby to grow.

4. If the mother has an inverted nipple
   a. the nursing baby is seldom precluded from suckling and obtaining milk.
   b. the breast does not function well; thus lactation should not be attempted.
   c. the breast produces milk, but the nipple does not function sufficiently to sustain the infant.
   d. breastfeeding proceeds more easily with the first baby than with later ones, for whom the inversion becomes more severe.

5. How the nipple looks when it emerges from the baby's mouth is
    a. w it should have looked when it first was grasped by the baby.
    b. how it should have looked when the baby was actively suckling.
    c. unrelated to how the nipple looks when not suckled.
    d. of importance only when the mother has inverted nipples.

6. Mastitis is usually characterized by
    a. a fever, slower-than-usual pulse, and inversion of the nipple on the affected side.
    b. bilateral tenderness and streaks moving from each nipple up the breast.
    c. a feeling that the breast is colder than usual.
    d. localized breast tenderness (usually unilateral), fatigue, and muscular aching.

7. A breast abscess
    a. is the outcome of approximately 90 percent of cases of mastitis.
    b. spells the end of breastfeeding on the affected side.
    c. will result in streptococcal bacteria in the breast.
    d. may require incision and drainage, after which breastfeeding can be resumed.

8. When a mother has eczema on the breasts and nipples, she
    a. must cease breastfeeding immediately to avoid infecting the baby.
    b. can be treated with a topical ointment.
    c. should make sure the baby is also treated to avoid continual cross-infection.
    d. will have to interrupt breastfeeding during the period of treatment.

9. Breast reduction or augmentation surgery will result in
    a. no effect on milk transfer if the mother has nonperiareolar surgery.
    b. low likelihood of sufficient milk transfer following periareolar surgery.
    c. no effect on milk transfer if the mother is a multip and has previously breastfed.
    d. no effect on milk transfer unless the mother gives birth prematurely.

10. Scarring caused by burns to the breast and nipple
    a. does not preclude breastfeeding.
    b. may be an indication of more severe internal trauma.
    c. nearly always means that the nipple pores have been destroyed.
    d. is a likely indicator of inadequate milk production.

Short-Answer Questions

1. Briefly discuss at least five recommendations for the treatment of a plugged duct.

2. Briefly discuss breast reduction surgery, noting when it is most likely to interfere with breast-feeding.

3. What is mastopexy and how is it done? Note whether it affects a woman's subsequent lactation course.

4. Briefly describe fibrocystic breast disease. How does it affect breastfeeding?

5. What is an intraductal papilloma? How is it identified, and what is its effect on subsequent lactation?

6. Briefly distinguish between infectious and noninfectious mastitis. In what ways would the treatment for the two differ?

7. What is a nipple blister?

8. Briefly define a nursing diagnosis, and indicate how it might be used to assist the lactation consultant in clinical practice.

9. Explain why breast surgery is viewed as a "double threat" to the woman experiencing it. What are such double threats?

10. Identify the different places where candidiasis/thrush can be found and what this means for the family in which more than one member exhibits symptoms.

11. Describe Raynaud's disease involving the nipples. How would you identify it, and what would be your recommended course of treatment so that the mother can continue breastfeeding?

12. Describe a breast lump that you suspect may be cancerous. What commonly occurring experiences during lactation could mirror the presentation of a tumor?

Essay Questions

1. What is the difference between breast augmentation and breast reduction surgery? In your discussion, distinguish between the two in terms of
    a. the woman's reaction to subsequent difficulty with breastfeeding.
    b. the likelihood of difficulty with breastfeeding.
    c. the nature of the surgery itself.

2. Discuss at least four factors that can contribute to development of mastitis. Indicate how each factor is related to the others and what you would recommend to assist the mother in resolving the problem.

3. How do you identify candidiasis/thrush in the baby's mouth? on the mother's breasts? In both cases, what is an appropriate remedy?

Story Problem

You feel assaulted by problems. In the past ten days, you've fielded questions and seen mothers with the following concerns: recurrent plugged ducts; mastitis; four cases of thrush; a breast abscess; one woman who wants to breastfeed following augmentation surgery; and three women who have had breast reduction surgery.

1. What do all of these women have in common?

2. Which of these women is least likely to be able to breastfeed completely?

3. Whom among this group have you asked to stop breastfeeding for two days in order to protect the baby?

4. In what sense do the mothers who have had surgery represent a problem of postindustrial society?

5. Following your visits with the women who have had reduction or augmentation surgery, what would you like for their cosmetic surgeons to know before they perform the same surgery on another woman in her childbearing years?

The woman with the recurrent plugged ducts asks you if her diet may have anything to do with her problems.

6. What is your reply?

She then asks what else she could be doing "wrong" that might be contributing to her difficulties.

7. After observing her baby at the breast, what is your answer to her question?

The phone rings; it's one of the clients with whom you worked for many weeks to clear up numerous early difficulties. She is tearful and confides, "I've found a lump in my breast – near my armpit. I'm scared to death. My mother died of breast cancer when I was 12. What should I do?"

8. Tell us your answer.

BEYOND POSTPARTUM

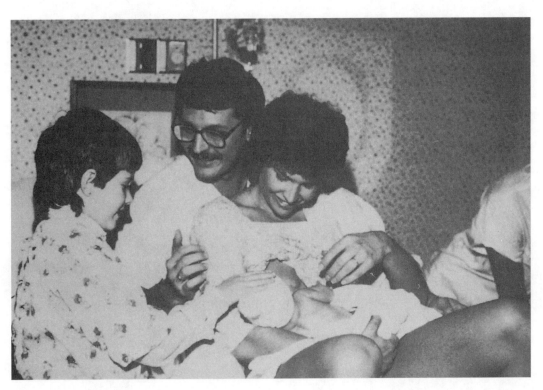

(Used with permission of Pat Bull.)

CHAPTER 16

Maternal Nutrition During Lactation

Outline

Key Concepts

You are urged to look for these key concepts in the body of the chapter and to develop questions deriving from these concepts as one way to gain understanding and insight into their relationship to lactation and breastfeeding. In this chapter, you are asked to consider how maternal nutrition affects the lactation course and the mother's milk production, and the most appropriate means by which to encourage optimal nutritional intake without placing undue emphasis on the need for "good nutrition."

Bone loss

Dietary intake

Dietary supplements

Fluid needs

Food flavoring

Food guide pyramid

Macronutrients

Maternal exercise

Maternal weight loss

Micronutrients

Multiple-Choice Questions

1. Which group of women takes in fewer calories during lactation?
    a. low-income African-American women
    b. affluent Caucasian women
    c. affluent African-American women
    d. only those on a highly restricted weight reduction program

2. Which of the following levels of food intake (measured in kcals) may result in an adverse effect on milk production?
    a. 2600 kcal/day
    b. 2200 kcal/day
    c. 1500 kcal/day
    d. 1000 kcal/day

3. What is the relationship between breastmilk calcium concentrations and maternal calcium intake?
    a. The more calcium the mother ingests, the higher the level of calcium in her milk.
    b. There is no relationship between breastmilk calcium levels and maternal calcium intake.
    c. The level of calcium in breastmilk is usually double that which the mother ingests.
    d. The level of calcium in breastmilk is usually half that which the mother ingests.

4. Which of the following is true regarding flavors in the maternal diet affecting breastmilk?
    a. Breastfed babies are less likely to accept solids because the flavors do not "match" the taste of the breastmilk they are used to.
    b. Breastfed babies tend to dislike highly flavored milk, particularly that which tastes like garlic.
    c. Breastfed babies tend to suckle longer and thus to obtain more milk when it is garlic flavored.
    d. Bottle-fed babies tend to be more accepting of solids because the flavors enhance the taste of the milk they have received for many weeks.

5. Weight loss during lactation is more likely to occur
    a. in the second six months of lactation.
    b. in the first six months of lactation.
    c. if the mother is a partial breastfeeder.
    d. after the mother has fully weaned her breastfeeding infant.

6. The lactating mother needs to drink
    a. at least four glasses of water daily.
    b. at least eight glasses of water daily.
    c. to thirst.
    d. twice as often as she breastfeeds the baby.

7. How many calories above her own needs should a mother be expected to use to maintain lactation?
    a. at least 1000 calories
    b. 750 to 1000 calories
    c. 500 to 750 calories
    d. 200 to 500 calories

Short-Answer Questions

1. What is the food guide pyramid? How should a mother use it?

2. What factors contribute to lactating women not taking in the RDAs expected?

3. Explain how metabolic efficiency during pregnancy and lactation may enable women to take in fewer calories without harm to themselves, their fetus, or their breastfeeding baby.

4. What would you advise a mother who wishes to begin a weight loss program when her baby is four weeks old?

5. Can exercise affect the lactating mother? In what ways? How can such exercise affect the breast-feeding baby?

6. Define three different classes of vegetarians. In what ways would their dietary restrictions influence your recommendations regarding seeking a balance of essential nutrients?

7. What do you tell pregnant mothers you meet at a corporate headquarters – sponsored session when they ask you about their coffee drinking while on the job? They want to know whether they will have to stop drinking coffee after their babies are born?

8. What are micronutrients? How might deficiencies in these elements manifest themselves?

Essay Questions

1. Examine the findings in Table 16-1. What conclusions you draw from the table findings? What would you recommend about daily caloric intake to a group of pregnant mothers? newly lactating women?

2. Consider the nutritional risk factors noted in Box 16-4. In each case, what would you recommend to a pregnant mother and to a breastfeeding mother in order to reduce the adverse effects of each of those risk factors?

3. Outline what you would tell women during pregnancy who are concerned about getting their weight "back to normal" (prepregnancy levels) as soon as possible after the birth of their babies. Include in your outline when these women can expect to lose weight, the effect of activity post-birth, and the influence of infant feeding patterns on such weight loss.

4. Review the outcome of studies examining the likelihood of bone loss in women due to infant feeding choice. How would these findings influence what you say to breastfeeding women concerned about the likelihood that they will develop osteoporosis later in life?

5. The Institute of Medicine recommends that breastfeeding women obtain all nutrients from food alone. A woman approaches you regarding which vitamin and mineral supplements she should continue following the birth of her baby. You learn that she is taking no fewer than seven different pills in addition to the food she is eating. What do you tell her?

6. In what ways are flavored foods a hint to the child about what to accept (or not) as food?

7. Define energy. How does this relate to BMR, caloric intake, weight gain/loss patterns, and need for dietary supplements by the "average" breastfeeding mother?

8. What are macronutrients? Include carbohydrates, protein, and fat in your answer and note how each is related to the other when creating an optimal food intake plan.

Story Problem

You're asked to offer a class focusing on nutrition to a group of women, half of whom are teenagers from a group home where they are living. The other half are women from a local advertising agency that has provided financial grants to the group home to enable it to continue offering a safe place for the teens to stay during their pregnancies.

1. What specific nutrient needs do these two groups of women represent?

2. One of the teens insists on drinking colas and eating candy during the class, to the acute discomfort of two of the advertising executives who are present. How do you dissuade her from continuing her insistence on high-sugar foods without appearing to "side with" the more affluent career women?

3. One of the corporate women asks how she can be expected to breastfeed when she plans to resume her weight-training and stair-climbing exercise regimen within two weeks of her baby's birth. She has been told by a friend that exercise "causes sour milk." What is your response?

4. You invite a former class member, now age 18, to return to the class with her baby, who weighed 7 pounds at birth. The baby is now five weeks old and already weighs 12 pounds. One of the women feels the baby's leg and points to her double chins and then exclaims, "This baby is obese! I will not allow my baby to get that big! If that is what breastfeeding does, I want no part of it!" The baby's mother is dismayed. What do you tell her? the rest of the class?

5. You are reviewing the food guide pyramid with the class. One of the teens complains that following it requires that she eat foods she cannot afford to buy. How do you respond?

6. Finally, during your last class session, you decide to review the seven recommendations provided by the U.S. dietary guidelines. Without alienating the rest of the people who are present, how do you counter the stage-whispered comments of two class members that no one is going to tell them how to eat or what to eat?

WOMEN'S HEALTH AND BREASTFEEDING

Outline

Key Concepts

You are urged to look for these key concepts in the body of the chapter and to develop questions deriving from these concepts as one way to gain you are asked to consider some of the implications of maternal illness on the lactation course and breastfeeding. In this chapter, you are asked to consider some of the implications of maternal illness on the lactation course and breastfeeding. Particularly helpful is a comparison between situations in which uneventful lactation is not an appropriate goal and situations in which maternal illness need not contraindicate the lactation course.

Asthma

Cystic fibrosis

Diabetes

Dysfunctional uterine bleeding

Endocrine functioning

Hyperthyroidism

Hypothyroidism

Impaired mobility

Induced lactation

Infections

Maternal smoking

Metabolic dysfunction

Multiple sclerosis

Pituitary dysfunction

Postpartum depression

Radioisotope studies

Relactation

Rheumatoid arthritis

Seizure disorder

Multiple-Choice Questions

1. A mother who experiences postpartum depression is likely to be a
   a. breastfeeding mother who would have preferred to bottle-feed.
   b. woman experiencing high levels of life stress with few supportive relationships.
   c. mother who is bottle-feeding.
   d. teen mother.

2. Insulin-dependent diabetes mellitus (IDDM) is
   a. an acute illness in the breastfeeding baby of the mother with diabetes.
   b. a chronic illness in the mother; she should be discouraged from breastfeeding.
   c. a chronic illness in the mother; she should be encouraged to breastfeed.
   d. an acute illness that can be treated with dietary changes alone.

3. Which of the following maternal conditions is likely to be reflected in poor weight gain in the baby?
   a. hypothyroidism
   b. hyperthyroidism
   c. diabetes mellitus
   d. prolactinoma

4. When a woman has cystic fibrosis, she
   a. should be strongly discouraged from breastfeeding.
   b. will produce milk that is insufficient to meet her baby's needs.
   c. needs close nutritional monitoring to maintain her own health.
   d. should not breastfeed because of the bacterial pathogens she carries.

5. When a mother has cystic fibrosis, breastfeeding can continue if the
   a. mother's weight declines.
   b. mother's health status is stable.
   c. mother's vitamin and caloric supplementation must be increased.
   d. mother is willing to give her baby formula as well.

6. When a mother has tuberculosis, she
   a. cannot breastfeed; to do so would endanger her baby.
   b. is unable to breastfeed; the illness precludes her from making milk.
   c. may breastfeed; separation from her infant is not necessary.
   d. may breastfeed, but will need to supplement her declining milk supply.

7. When a mother must have surgery, she should be encouraged to
   a. breastfeed as soon after the surgery as possible.
   b. begin pumping her breasts 12 hours before surgery, and for 36 hours postsurgery.
   c. breastfeed before the surgery and then pump her breasts for the first week postsurgery.
   d. wean the baby in advance of the surgery to make her life less stressful.

8. Relactation is easier if the baby
   a. is at least three months old and thus stronger than a newborn.
   b. is willing to share the breast with an older breastfeeding toddler.
   c. has previously been bottle-fed and thus needs lots of cuddling.
   d. enjoys breastfeeding and is willing to do so frequently.

Short-Answer Questions

1. What is the difference between an acute and a chronic illness? Select one example of each.

2. Briefly discuss the relationship between weight loss and maternal exercise during lactation.

3. What is a prolactinoma? How does it influence lactation?

4. What is a self-limiting illness? Briefly explain how antibiotic therapy for such an illness will affect the breastfeeding baby of a mother receiving such therapy.

5. Explain how excessive bleeding in the postpartum period can negatively affect the lactation course.

6. Briefly explain why one cannot predict whether/when an adoptive breastfeeding mother will develop a milk supply sufficient to completely nourish the breastfeeding baby. Refer to at least one maternal and one infant factor in your answer.

7. What is multiple sclerosis? How does it affect the mother choosing to breastfeed? Her breastfeeding baby?

8. Briefly explain how a mother might avoid exposing her baby to radioactive isotopes following a diagnostic study requiring their use.

9. Briefly outline what foods you would encourage a breastfeeding mother to eat and which she should avoid if she is concerned about losing excess weight she gained before she became pregnant and maintaining sufficient energy to make "good" milk for her baby.

10. Briefly discuss at least five recommendations you would make to a mother with limited mobility. In each case, indicate your reason for offering such a recommendation.

11. Explain why a mother who has breastfed babies born to her may enjoy breastfeeding an adopted baby less than a woman who has never been able to have children.

Essay Questions

1. A mother with a history of epilepsy asks how she might make her home safe for her baby in the event she has a seizure. What do you suggest to her? Why?

2. What is SLE? How does it affect the lactation course?

3. Distinguish between relactation and induced lactation. Identify at least two benefits of these lactation options and two potentially negative consequences.

4. From a hormonal perspective, what is the normal postpartum state? How does this relate to postpartum depression? to usual treatment regimens? to the mother's plan to breastfeed?

5. Indicate how nicotine addiction influences milk production and the breastfeeding infant. What is the most appropriate recommendation to make to a nicotine-addicted mother regarding breastfeeding prior to her baby's birth?

6. What is the linkage between headaches and breastfeeding? How might you assist the mother who suffers from migraine headaches and doesn't want to end her breastfeeding relationship before her baby is ready to do so?

Story Problem

You're part of a private practice only recently affiliated with a major medical center. You've been asked to speak to a group of residents in internal medicine about breastfeeding during maternal illness.

1. Outline the portion of your talk that focuses the residents' attention on the normal course of lactation for the healthy mother.

2. Distinguish among the healthy, the acutely ill, and the chronically ill mother who wishes to breastfeed. Justify the distinctions you've made and those elements that need not be different for the mother with an illness.

In the midst of your presentation, a hand is raised in the back of the room. Your host has warned you in advance of your presentation that the department chair is from "the old school." She doesn't believe that breastfeeding is safe if the mother is on any kind of drug. You suspect that the distinguished-looking older woman waving her hand is the chair. She asks, "What about the mother taking medications?"

3. Outline your answer, making sure that you include a response that includes medications used to treat an acute illness, a chronic illness, postpartum depression, and following a radioisotope scan. Note: The choice of illness in each case is yours!

The same hand waves again. "It sounds to me like you're saying... Is that right?"

4. Tell us what the physician has said to you. How do you make her interpretation of your comments more accurate?

Your lecture is over. Several residents approach you during the break between lectures. One tells you his sister is adopting a baby and wants to breastfeed. He wants some advice he can give her when he sees her over the New Year holidays.

5. What do you ask him before replying to his question?

6. What information do you offer that he can take home to his sister?

Another resident calls you at your office a few days after the lecture. She has a breastfeeding patient whom she has treated for asthma. She now suspects that this patient has returned to smoking, a behavior that the resident had strongly discouraged. The patient is worried about her baby's behavior, which includes colic. The pediatrician has offered "relaxing drops" for the baby, which the mother is not comfortable with. The resident wants to know if it is possible for the baby to be reacting to the mother's smoking.

7. How do you respond?

Maternal Employment and Breastfeeding

Outline

Key Concepts

You are urged to look for these key concepts in the body of the chapter and to develop questions deriving from these concepts as one way to gain understanding and insight into their relationship to lactation and breastfeeding. In this chapter, you are asked to consider how paid employment outside the home alters women's plans for themselves and their babies and how those plans can continue to include breastfeeding. In some cases, comparing the at-home mother with her neighbor who leaves for work each morning might highlight specific clinical concerns designed to assist the employed breastfeeding mother.

Bottle-feeding

Breast pumping

Cup-feeding

Day-care

Expressing milk

Fatigue

Maternity leave

Milk storage

Prenatal planning

"Reverse cycle nursing"

Social support

Spoon-feeding

The "5-15-5" rule

Multiple-Choice Questions

1. All of the following are reasons mothers express milk when they are regularly separated from their babies, EXCEPT
   a. to remain physically comfortable on the job.
   b. to reduce the likelihood of leaking while on the job.
   c. to collect milk for immediate use by the baby.
   d. to collect milk for later use by the baby.

2. "Reverse cycle nursing" refers to
   a. altering the cycling pattern of a breast pump in order to increase the pressure it exerts on the breast.
   b. the baby who sleeps more in the mother's absence and is more wakeful when she is available.
   c. the mother who changes her pattern of breastfeeding at home to mimic that which occurs when she is at work.
   d. An alteration in the pattern of breastfeeding that serves to reduce the mother's milk supply so that she need not express milk when separated from the baby.

3. Job-sharing refers to
   a. what a husband does when he works at home full time and his wife works outside the home full time.
   b. when two individuals work part-time in the same position, as opposed to one employee who works full time in the same position.
   c. what happens when an employee does part of her work at home and part of her work at work.
   d. when the husband shares the home work that his wife has previously assumed as her responsibility.

4. Spoon-feeding liquids to an infant is possible
   a. once the baby is able to sit up unaided.
   b. when the baby can be safely propped into a highchair.
   c. when the baby is at least two months old.
   d. from birth onward.

5. When selecting a day-care facility, the parents should consider ALL BUT ONE of the following:
    a   the experiences of previous users of the facility
    b. the cleanliness and safety features of the facility
    c. opportunities for numerous kinds of learning
    d. the frequency with which physician visits are made

6. Mothers who view breastfeeding positively are inclined to
    a. breastfeed longer, even if they are employed.
    b. select home care settings rather than group day care for their babies.
    c. delay until six months their return to work, in order to stay with their babies.
    d. decide not to return to work following their baby's birth.

Short-Answer Questions

1. Briefly distinguish between different day-care settings, noting the positive and negative aspects of each setting.

2. Briefly offer at least three recommendations the employed mother may wish to consider when she plans to store her expressed milk for later use.

3. Identify at least four questions a mother should ask if she is planning to use a breast pump.

4. Identify at least three illnesses that are apt to occur when an infant or young child is cared for outside his or her own home. In each case, note whether breastfeeding is likely to reduce its incidence or severity.

5. Identify five different individuals who can serve as a source of social support for the employed breastfeeding mother. In each case, provide an example of what they can do to help the person they are serving.

6. Explain the difference between the length of a breast pumping experience and the duration of specific pumping sessions when seeking to obtain optimal breastmilk for later feedings. How would you recommend that a mother express or pump her milk in order to obtain as much milk as possible?

7. Explain the "5-15-5" rule and how it relates to maintaining physical comfort on the job.

8. When is the mother most likely to experience each of the following, and what would you recommend to her in order to avoid or reduce each item's effect on her upon her return to work?
    a. engorgement and/or leaking
    b. the baby's frequent changes of feeding patterns
    c. concern about an inadequate or fluctuating milk supply
    d. the need to express or pump milk

9. Explain why the nature of the mother's work, the baby's age, and the type of support the mother has (and from whom) can influence whether and how long she feels she is able to combine breastfeeding with employment.

Essay Questions

1. Using the following issues, explain to a colleague how you will assist a breastfeeding mother who has returned to work and does not want to use any artificial baby milk. Compare your recommendation in that situation to one in which the mother does not plan to express her milk, even when she is at home. In each case, touch on the five elements listed below:
   a. When will she return to work?
   b. How long will she breastfeed?
   c. Will she express or pump milk?
   d. Will she give her baby artificial baby milk for missed feedings?
   e. Where will the baby be cared for?

2. Identify at least four barriers to breastfeeding after returning to paid employment. In each case, indicate how each barrier can be reduced or eliminated so that it no longer serves as a reason for not breastfeeding.

3. Briefly discuss the issues involved in the timing of a breastfeeding woman's return to work – including her total work hours/week and projected breastfeeding duration. What would you recommend to an employed breastfeeding mother who wishes to continue breastfeeding longer than six months?

4. Review the following four case presentations.

   Situation A: Mary Smith gave birth yesterday. She wonders aloud whether she should breastfeed. She knows she will be returning to her part-time job (four hours a day, five days a week) when the baby is six weeks old. Her two other children, now four and seven years old, respectively, were bottle-fed. She said in her childbirth class that she wanted to nurse this, her last, baby.

   Situation B: Sharnelle Johnson is returning to full-time work as a warehouse and packing employee when her firstborn is four weeks old. She just got her job last month and needs to return to it as soon as her maternity leave is over. She works eight hours a day, five days a week; her travel time to and from work is 30 minutes. Her mother, who bottle-fed all nine of her children, has agreed to watch Sharnelle's daughter for her. On the job, she operates a forklift and does some manual lifting as well. All her coworkers are men.

   Situation C: Debbie Andersen is going back to finish her junior year in high school three months after giving birth. She says she wants to breastfeed; it is now her third day postpartum and she and the baby are doing well.

   Situation D: Joan Gilbert has taken a 10-week leave from her private pediatric practice after the birth of her second baby. Her husband is completing law school this year. Joan nursed her first baby for eight weeks before discovering that her patients' needs were more intrusive than she had expected.

For each of the above case studies, answer the following questions:
   a. What additional information do you need?
   b. What will you tell her about (1) breastfeeding; (2) being a new parent; (3) continuing to breastfeed after returning to work or school; (4) child behavior in the first year?
   c. What, specifically, does this new mother need to know about combining breastfeeding and working or going to school?

d. How might others (grandparents, spouse, friends, coworkers) help her? How likely is this to happen?

e. If this is not her first breastfeeding experience, how might she breastfeed longer than she did previously?

f. If she has not breastfed before, what does she need to know about how breastfeeding and breastfed babies are different from bottle-feeding and bottle-fed babies?

g. What particular elements about her work or school situation are apt to be most troublesome regarding her baby's needs and her breastfeeding experience?

h. Should she even bother to breastfeed?

I. How can you help her to have a positive breastfeeding experience?

Story Problem

Joan Williams is planning to return to work after her baby's birth. She has asked for a prenatal consultation so that her baby's presence will not interfere with her career plans.

1. How do you respond to her questions?

One of your colleagues overhears Joan's questions and quips, "Good luck! There's no baby alive who's ever taken into account his mother's career plans!" Joan bursts into tears.

2. What do you say to Joan? to your colleague?

Joan's baby is born following a 35-hour labor which culminates in an assisted vaginal birth, resulting in moderate to severe blood loss and severe tearing of the perineum. At three weeks postpartum, Joan is still complaining about her hemorrhoid pain, tiredness, and nipple tenderness. Her baby cries a great deal, and Joan is tired of taking the additional iron pills her doctor has prescribed. She plans to return to work next week and wants your advice.

3. What do you tell her?

Joan calls you from the office two days after returning to work. She is crying. "What am I going to do?" she sobs. "I can barely walk, much less run up and down stairs all day. I went into a big meeting and leaked all over the front of my blouse when one of my bosses asked about the baby. And Jason kept me up all last night wanting to nurse. Every time I tried to put him down, he cried and fussed. I'm exhausted – and it's only 2 o'clock! I have to be here for at least another three hours!"

4. What is your reply?

Joan calls in sick the next two days and goes to bed with the baby. She forgets to take the iron pills and finds that she is less gassy and the baby is less fussy. "Is there a connection there?" she asks.

5. How do you reply? What explanation do you give her?

Two months later, Joan calls you asking for referral for a new babysitter. She is unhappy with the current sitter; her husband thinks she is simply unhappy having to leave the baby for ten hours a day. She reports having asked the sitter to use a cup rather than a bottle to feed the baby. The sitter contends that the baby will choke and she will not be responsible!

6. What is your response?

CHILD HEALTH

Outline

Key Concepts

You are urged to look for these key concepts in the body of the chapter and to develop questions deriving from these concepts as one way to gain understanding and insight into their relationship to lactation and breastfeeding. You are asked to pay particular attention to normal growth and development and to how the experience of breastfeeding relates to such growth.

Arousal

Attachment

Communication

Dental health

Habituation

Immunization

Nature vs. nurture

Obesity

Reflexes

Senses

Separation

Social development

Stranger distress

Temperament

Weaning

Multiple-Choice Questions

1. Asking a 6- to 12-month old child to engage in "time out" behavior in his room
   a. is appropriate for this age group.
   b. is more appropriate for a younger child.
   c. is more appropriate for an older child.
   d. can be taught at any time; it is unrelated to the child's age and developmental stage.

2. Weaning that occurs rapidly may require that the mother
   a. express or pump her breasts to reduce fullness.
   b. avoid holding the baby lest he ask to nurse.
   c. use cold showers to reduce the likelihood of breast leakage.
   d. obtain an antibiotic in advance should mastitis occur.

3. Immunization of breastfed children
   a. should be delayed until after weaning from the breast to assure that the immunization "takes."
   b. usually results in a higher antibody level than in artificially fed children.
   c. should be repeated after weaning to verify that the immunization "took."
   d. should be avoided in order to eliminate theoretical adverse reaction to the immunization medium.

4. In the first year, a baby's
   a. weight usually doubles.
   b. weight usually triples.
   c. length usually increases by 50 percent.
   d. length usually increases by 100 percent.

5. Motor development progresses from _____ to _____.
   a. small muscle control, large muscle control
   b. feet and legs, arms and head
   c. large muscle control, small muscle control
   d. arms and legs, head and neck

6. The infant can best maintain complex interactions with his environment in the
   a. quiet alert state.
   b. soft crying state.
   c. hard crying state.
   d. restless awake state.

Short-Answer Questions

1. Distinguish between five different states of arousal. Which state is optimal for breastfeeding? Why is this?

2. Briefly distinguish between Erikson's and Piaget's views of a toddler. Use at least two different elements to support your view.

3. Identify three different factors that have been related to childhood obesity. In what way is breastfeeding related to these factors?

4. Briefly discuss three developmental cues that infer readiness for solid foods.

5. Briefly discuss the phases of response that occur when a mother or father leaves a young child with strangers. Indicate ways in which a lactation consultant might interact with such a child without triggering "stranger anxiety."

6. How does a baby sleep? What implications does this have for the breastfeeding course?

7. Briefly distinguish between receptive and expressive language.

8. Define habituation. Give an example.

9. What is meant by cephalocaudal and proximaldistal growth?

10. What is motherese and why is it significant to the infant's interaction?

Essay Questions

1. Discuss four reflexes that are most likely to be present in the first few months of an infant's life. In each case indicate how the reflex relates to breastfeeding behavior.

2. Characterize an "easy" child, a "slow-to-warm-up" child, and a "difficult" child, and provide a breastfeeding-related example, with regard to each of the following factors:
   a. adapting to a change in routine
   b. a positive or negative mood
   c. attention span
   d. distractability
   e. sensory threshold

3. Infant behaviors, including those related to breastfeeding, change over time. Select five different ages. For each age period indicate at least three typical behaviors of a child that age, including one related to breastfeeding.

4. Explain why solid foods should be delayed until the second half of the first year of life.

5. Attachment has been discussed as a process in which both parent and child participate. Discuss how a baby cues a parent to engage in appropriate nurturing behavior. Discuss how a parent cues a baby to be appropriately responsive.

6. Describe the many ways in which infant growth occurs through the first year. Include in your description weight, height, and developmental changes.

7. Discuss Bowlby's findings relating to "hospitalism" and Ainsworth's examination of secure and insecure attachment behaviors. How are these two studies related to our understanding of the bonding/attachment process?

Story Problem

You are asked to teach a growth and development class to high school sophomores.

1. Indicate how you would illustrate how a baby grows.

2. Relate such growth to feeding behavior.

A student asks you to distinguish between the importance of nature and of nurture in producing a healthy child who grows to healthy adulthood.

3. Do so.

One student protests, "But you never mentioned formula-feeding. Does that mean that my mother, who formula-fed me, didn't provide a healthy environment?"

4. How do you answer her question?

Another student asks you if rooming-in is all that important, especially because women stay in hospitals for such a short time today: "Wouldn't it just be better if they got as much rest as possible and worried about the baby when they got home?"

5. How do you respond to his concerns?

The last question from the class relates to dental health and breastfeeding.

6. How do you respond to the teacher's request that you define nursing-bottle caries and how breastfed babies are at risk for this problem?

THE ILL BREASTFEEDING CHILD

Outline

Key Concepts

You are urged to look for these key concepts in the body of the chapter and to develop questions deriving from these concepts as one way to gain understanding and insight into their relationship to lactation and breastfeeding. In this chapter, you are asked to compare the breastfeeding course of a healthy infant with that of one who is ill. You can gain insight by distinguishing between an infant with an acute illness and an infant with a chronic condition. You should also pay attention to how infant illness affects the lactation course and parenting patterns.

Allergies

Celiac disease

Choanal atresia

Cleft lip/palate

Congenital heart defects

Congenital hypothyroidism

Cystic fibrosis

Down syndrome

Esophageal reflux

Galactosemia

Gastrointestinal infection

Grief

Hospitalization

Hydrocephalus

Hypoglycemia

Imperforate anus

Inborn errors of metabolism

"Magic milk" syndrome

Meningitis

Myelomeningocele

Otitis media

Pyloric stenosis

Respiratory infection

Sudden infant death syndrome (SIDS)

Tracheoesophageal fistula

Multiple-Choice Questions

1. Treatment for slight to mild dehydration from gastroenteritis in breastfeeding infants includes
   a. continued breastfeeding and replacement fluids if necessary.
   b. interrupted breastfeeding and breast pumping during the acute phase of the illness.
   c. continued breastfeeding and formula supplements.
   d. hospitalization with intravenous fluids and electrolytes.

2. Sudden infant death syndrome
   a. is most often a missed infanticide.
   b. never occurs in breastfeeding babies.
   c. is usually a diagnosis that is unconfirmed until autopsy.
   d. is usually followed by mastitis.

3. What is the number of wet cloth diapers expected within a 24-hour period in a breastfeeding infant?
   a. two to four
   b. three to six
   c. four to seven
   d. six to eight

4. Which of the following is a contraindication to breastfeeding by an affected infant?
   a. galactosemia
   b. cystic fibrosis
   c. PKU
   d. celiac disease

5. Which of the following is an indication of dehydration?
   a. normal anterior fontanel but depressed posterior fontanel
   b. dry mucous membranes
   c. very warm extremities
   d. low grade fever

6. Excessive fluid loss in an infant occurs most often
   a. from frequent vomiting.
   b. from urination.
   c. through the skin.
   d. from stooling.

7. When a baby is born with a cleft lip and palate, the usual repair plan is
   a. palate first if unilateral, then the lip.
   b. lip first, then the palate.
   c. lip first and, if bilateral, the anterior portion of the palate, followed by the posterior portion of the palate.
   d. lip and palate are usually repaired at the same time to avoid a second surgery.

Short-Answer Questions

1. Briefly identify at least five different foods that are associated with allergic reactions in infants or young children. Indicate foods in which they are most likely to be found.

2. Briefly discuss the rationale behind very early repair of a cleft lip. Include in your answer such factors as length of hospital stay, weight gain, and consideration of the repair site.

3. What is rotavirus, and how does breastfeeding reduce its likelihood of consequences for the infant?

4. Briefly explain why oral glucose water should not be given to the hypoglycemic neonate.

5. Distinguish between food allergy, food intolerance, and food sensitivity.

6. What is celiac disease, and how is it related to infant feeding patterns?

7. What is congenital hypothyroidism? How might breastfeeding alter the course of the disease?

8. What is phenylketonuria, and how is it related to breastfeeding?

9. Outline ways to prepare a young child for surgery. In what ways might such preparation be different for a baby or young child receiving human milk?

10. Briefly explain how the "dancer hand" position might assist a mother who is breastfeeding an ill infant or young child.

11. Upper respiratory illnesses can affect a baby's desire to feed. Briefly explain what is meant by this statement and what you might tell a mother whose baby has such an illness.

Essay Questions

1. Identify at least five principles of care during the hospitalization of a baby with a serious respiratory illness.

2. Explain how hospitalization can disrupt the life experience of a breastfeeding family. Indicate how such disruption can be minimized.

3. Your client's baby has been diagnosed with cystic fibrosis at 15 months of age – two months after weaning completely from the breast. What do you tell her when she asks if breastfeeding had anything to do with the baby's disease?

4. Identify each of the following problems and discuss how it relates to oral feedings generally and to breastfeeding specifically:
   a. choanal atresia
   b. cleft palate
   c. tracheoesophageal fistula (T-E fistula)
   d. pyloric stenosis
   e. imperforate anus
   f. esophageal reflux

5. Explain how breastfeeding may be affected when a child is born with each of the following conditions:
   a. Down syndrome
   b. hydrocephalus
   c. myelomeningocele
   d. congenital heart defect

6. What is GE reflux and how does it affect the breastfeeding mother and baby?

7. Explain why cow milk allergy is the most common nutritional allergy during infancy.

Story Problem

The city where you live is experiencing an epidemic of upper respiratory illness, sometimes requiring hospitalization. Few of your breastfeeding clients have reported that their breastfeeding infants have been affected.

1. How do you explain this phenomenon to a class of pregnant couples who have expressed concern about giving birth in the midst of this epidemic?

One of your clients calls and asks if you feel she should bring her baby to the doctor. The child has refused to nurse and seems lethargic. In all other respects he seems normal to the mother.

2. What is your response to her?

Another one of your clients has just given birth to a baby with Down syndrome.

3. What do you tell her about the baby's ability to breastfeed when she asks if she can continue to feed her as she has her other five children?

A sick baby is seen by his doctor, who immediately admits him to the pediatric unit of the local hospital. The mother calls you, distraught that the nurses on the unit assume he is bottle-fed and are upset that he has refused to accept a bottle.

4. What do you advise the mother?

At the mother's insistence, a nurse from the hospital calls you. It is clear from her tone that she is contacting you under duress and would prefer not to be involved.

5. What do you tell her about this mother and her three-month-old infant who is exclusively breast-fed?

The baby in question has been placed in a croupette to assist his breathing. When you see the mother, she is exhausted from worry and is unable to sleep on the foldout chair that is in the baby's room. Her husband just called for news about the baby; during their conversation he mentions that their two older children, one of whom is a preschooler, are very upset at their mother's absence.

6. How do you help the mother to feel able to cope with her simultaneous desire to remain with her baby and her guilt at not being with her other children?

7. How do you help her to manage some of the difficulties of continued milk production in the face of her baby's distress and disinterest in breastfeeding; her increasingly full breasts; her difficulty expressing milk using a hand pump with a bulb syringe that the nurses have provided her; and her general exhaustion?

The mother's baby has been in the hospital for four days. On the first night the mother chooses not to stay at the hospital with her baby, he dies suddenly.

8. When her husband calls to tell you this, what four suggestions do you offer to help this family cope with their grief and loss? In your answer, be sure to discuss what you might share with the parents about how to help each other, as well as their remaining children.

9. Following receipt of this family's letter to the hospital administrator questioning several aspects of the care their child received during his illness, you are asked to present an in-service to the emergency room staff about how to manage a breastfeeding mother and baby when one is admitted to their service. Outline what you will share with them and why you have decided to focus on each of the recommendations you plan to offer.

21

FERTILITY, SEXUALITY, AND CONTRACEPTION DURING LACTATION

Outline

Key Concepts

You are urged to look for these key concepts in the body of the chapter and to develop questions deriving from these concepts as one way to gain understanding and insight into their relationship to lactation and breastfeeding. In this chapter in particular, you are cautioned to consider each concept from at least two perspectives: both in the absence of lactation and during lactation. In some cases, insight into the concept can also be gained by comparing the prepregnancy period with the postbirth period.

Amenorrhea

Contraception

Family planning

Fertility

Intercourse
Libido
Ovulation patterns
Sexuality
Supplemental feeding

Multiple-Choice Questions

1. When a mother breastfeeds at least seven times daily, ovulation is prevented from occurring.
   a. True; in exclusively breastfeeding mothers the frequency of suckling prevents ovulation.
   b. False; even in exclusively breastfeeding mothers the frequency of suckling does not prevent ovulation.
   c. True; ovulation is especially unlikely in the second six months of the child's life when frequent suckling occurs.
   d. False; only in nutritionally at-risk mothers will frequent suckling stimulation inhibit ovulation.

2. The Bellagio consensus contends that exclusive breastfeeding provides
   a. more than 75 percent protection against pregnancy during the second six months postpartum.
   b. more than 75 percent protection against pregnancy during the first six months postpartum.
   c. more than 98 percent protection against pregnancy during the first six months postpartum.
   d. less than 15 percent protection against pregnancy during the second six months postpartum.

3. In many developed countries, frequency of sexual intercourse _____ following the birth of a baby
   a. declines over time.
   b. increases over time.
   c. declines and then increases.
   d. increases and then declines.

4. Which of the following <u>delays</u> first ovulation and subsequent risk of pregnancy?
   a. infrequent infant suckling
   b. daily duration of infant suckling
   c. supplementation of the infant's diet with nonhuman milk foods/fluids
   d. pacifier use

5. Vaginal bleeding in the breastfeeding woman in the early weeks following birth
   a. indicates that her menses have returned.
   b. can usually be ignored unless it is very heavy.
   c. indicates that ovulation has occurred.
   d. indicates she has resumed intercourse too soon.

6. Ideal timing for the use of progestin-only contraceptives, without adversely affecting the early breastfeeding course, is
   a. within 72 hours of delivery.
   b. prior to hospital discharge.
   c. after 6 weeks postpartum.
   d. after 12 weeks postpartum.

7. Counseling for family planning is ideally provided
    a. before delivery with postpartum followup timed to match the method chosen.
    b. immediately after delivery, with followup within the first two weeks postpartum.
    c. after hospital discharge, with followup at the six-week visit.
    d. after six weeks postpartum, following verification that breastfeeding is going well.

Short-Answer Questions

1. Identify at least one permanent and one nonpermanent method of nonhormonal contraception and two methods of hormonal contraception.

2. What is the lactational amenorrhea method (LAM) of contraception?

3. What is "silent ovulation," and how might one suspect that it has occurred during lactation?

4. Briefly explain the effect of suckling stimulus on
    a. the maintenance of milk production.
    b. inhibition of ovulation.
    c. milk ejection.

5. Explain why menses is considered an "absolute indication" of the need for a contraceptive method if another baby is not desired at this time.

6. Distinguish between pregnancy prevention and child spacing.

7. Briefly explain the role of the following in the normal menstrual course of a nonlactating woman:
    a. GnRH
    b. luteinizing hormone (LH)

8. How are levels of LH changed in a lactating woman compared to a woman who is not producing milk for a suckling infant?

Essay Questions

1. What is the relationship between contraception, fertility, sexuality, and lactation?

2. Discuss the risks and benefits of at least five different contraceptive methods during the lactation course. In each case, identify at least one risk and one benefit to the lactating mother and her breastfeeding infant when such a method of contraception is used.

3. Identify which method of contraception you would recommend in each of the following situations. Justify your answer in each case.
    a. A woman of color, age 15, who has never used contraception in the past and who gave birth to an infant who died yesterday, 22 days after birth.
    b. A woman with two living children, ages 13 months and 2 weeks, respectively. She is married and her husband strenuously objects to using condoms.
    c. A woman with a newborn infant who is currently breastfeeding 12 or more times daily. This mother previously used an oral contraceptive but is hesitant to do so while she is lactating.

    d. A woman with a one-month-old infant. Her religious affiliation precludes limiting the number of children born to her and her mate. Although she is fearful that her children will be born "too close" together, she is reluctant to use a method of contraception that is "obvious."

    e. A mother with her fifth child, the last two of whom are only 15 months apart. The mother has breastfed all her children and intends to do so with her new baby as well. She fears having another pregnancy because of financial problems and concerns about how she will house and clothe her family.

4. Compare the implications of male versus female sterilization for the family happy to have two children and no more.

Story Problem

Yolanda is 22 years old; she had her first child six weeks ago. Manuel, the father of her baby, is thrilled to be a new father and has already expressed his desire for more children. Yolanda is breastfeeding and wants more children – "but not right away."

1. How do you address Yolanda's partner's desire for more children while supporting Yolanda's wish not to get pregnant quickly?

2. What methods of birth control/child spacing would you discuss with these new parents? Why would you choose these methods to discuss?

In the course of your discussion, you learn that Yolanda's partner has been pressuring her to have intercourse. However, the first time they did so after the baby's birth, Yolanda experienced a great deal of pain. She offered to help him have an orgasm but refused to allow him to penetrate her vagina.

3. What would you tell them about intercourse in the early postpartum period?

4. How would you counter Manuel's conclusion that Yolanda's breastfeeding is making intercourse painful for her?

Yolanda wants to use condoms and a spermicidal foam/jelly; Manuel does not. He prefers that Yolanda go on the pill if she <u>must</u> protect against pregnancy until their baby is a bit older.

5. How would you help them to see which of these choices may be appropriate for Yolanda while she is breastfeeding?

6. What other factors would you raise as they consider the risks and benefits of these methods of contraception?

7. Sexual feelings in the postpartum period reflect many aspects of parenthood. What information should you share with Yolanda about her own psyche and body responses – and those of her partner – in order to help her understand why their responsiveness may differ from their sexual expression prior to parenthood?

Manuel wants Yolanda to stop breastfeeding. He doesn't trust that she won't become pregnant – even when they are using "something else."

8. What do you need to know about Yolanda's lactation course and the baby's breastfeeding behavior in order to assess how likely Yolanda is to become pregnant
    a. when her baby is less than three months old?
    b. when her baby is between four and six months old?
    c. when her baby is more than six months old?

CONTEMPORARY ISSUES

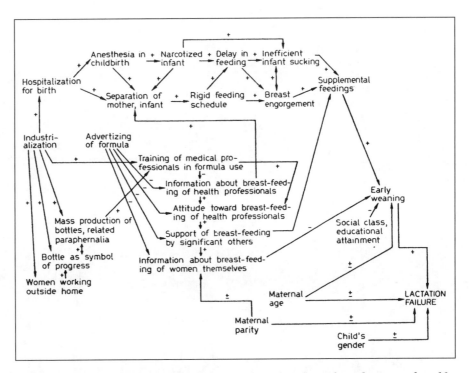

From Figure 1, Auerbach KG: The ecological, clinical, and sociological aspects of world-wide lactation failure, pp. 415–418; in Hirsch H, ed: The Family, Fourth International Congress of Psychosomatic Obstetrics and Gynecology, Tel Aviv, 1974 (Karger:Basel 1975).

WORK STRATEGIES AND THE LACTATION CONSULTANT

Outline

History

Certification

Educational offerings

Hospital lactation programs

Playing politics

The unique characteristics of breastfeeding counseling

Assertiveness

Roles and responsibilities

Lactation Consultants and voluntary counselors

Marketing

Networking

   Reporting and charting

   Nursing diagnosis

   Methods for charting

Clinical care plans

Legal considerations

Reimbursements

The LC in hospital-based practice

The LC in private practice

The business of doing business

Collaboration with other health care workers

Partnerships

Burnout

Do's and don'ts of lactation consulting

Key Concepts

You are urged to look for these key concepts in the body of the chapter and to develop questions deriving from these concepts as one way to gain understanding and insight into their relationship to lactation and breastfeeding. In this chapter, your attention is called to the similarities in development between lactation consultation as an allied health profession and the medical profession – which also developed out of a mentoring and apprenticeship form of training in advance of the availability of formalized academic training at a university. The reader may wish to compare the activities of lactation consultants with those of other health care workers, noting both the commonalities and those areas where divergences occur.

Assertiveness

Burnout

Cash flow

Certification

Charting

Hospital privileges

Lactation consulting

Legal liability

Partnership

Politics

Rounds

Multiple-Choice Questions

1. When working with women coworkers, it is best to
   a. be friendly, but not a best friend with coworkers.
   b. remain aloof from coworkers.
   c. keep track of and report their mistakes to the supervisor.
   d. expect your coworkers not to support you.

2. State licensure
   a. is governed by an agency of the federal government.
   b. prohibits nonlicensed individuals from legally practicing the trade in question.
   c. infers a minimum level of professional competence from licensed individuals.
   d. enables nonlicensed individuals to practice if they are certified or registered.

3. A health care provider who is supportive of lactation services usually
   a. has observed or has had a positive breastfeeding experience.
   b. is a medical school graduate from the 1940s or 1950s.
   c. has a well-established practice and thus can "experiment" with something new.
   d. has gained most of his or her breastfeeding knowledge from commercial milk companies.

4. The history of lactation consulting reveals that it
   a. developed when physicians recognized that its time-intensive nature was more than they could provide.
   b. developed when licensing boards recognized that certification was a more appropriate avenue to assess minimal competency.
   c. developed out of the voluntary assistance provided by women to other women who sought to offer care within, as well as adjunct to, other health care services.
   d. developed out of recognition of need demanded by patients and subsequently governmentally mandated.

5. In the past decade, hospitals have increasingly required that the LC be
   a. certified by the IBLCE.
   b. licensed as an M.D. or D.O.
   c. directly supervised by an M.D. on staff.
   d. a member of a team of similarly trained individuals.

6. Which of the following statements is true concerning the IBCLE examination?
   a. The number of candidates has declined over the years.
   b. The pass-fail score has increased in recent years.
   c. The percentage of passing candidates has gradually declined over time.
   d. The mean scores of passing candidates is in the 70s.

7. Symptoms of burnout include
   a. recognition that you are one of several experts who can help breastfeeding mothers.
   b. willingness to work as a team member.
   c. feeling cynical and/or frustrated with your job.
   d. knowing that everyone appreciates your assistance with breastfeeding women.

Short-Answer Questions

1. Briefly distinguish between a lactation consultant and a voluntary breastfeeding counselor.

2. Define assertiveness as it is used in this chapter. Briefly note how it differs from aggressiveness as a means of reaching a goal or solving a problem.

3. Identify the target audience for each of the following potential referral sources. Note which group is most likely to be the best advertisement and why.
   a. physicians
   b. mothers
   c. office nurses
   d. the general community

4. Distinguish between a solo practice and a partnership by noting five differences between the two.

5. What elements of a hospital-based lactation program can also be engaged in by an LC in private practice? Which elements should be limited to a hospital-based program?

6. Define burnout. Offer an example of how it can occur.

7. Identify three problems relating to private lactation consulting. Indicate how each might be resolved or prevented from occurring in the first place.

8. Briefly discuss each of the following legal issues. Include in your discussion an example that clearly avoids the legal problem in question.
   a. permission to touch
   b. avoiding a guarantee
   c. avoiding causing emotional distress
   d. confidentiality of information

9. Outline how in-hospital LCs and private practice LCs can work together to provide complete, long-term services to breastfeeding mothers in the community.

Essay Questions

1. What is problem-oriented medical record-keeping? Provide a brief example focusing on some aspect of breastfeeding. Indicate at least two different ways in which this method of charting can serve
   a. when the LC works in a physician's office.
   b. when the LC works in a hospital.
   c. when the LC maintains a private practice.

2. Identify four advantages and four disadvantages to incorporation for a practice in lactation consulting. In each case, note how an advantage might become a disadvantage and how a disadvantage might be changed into an advantage.

3. Read Table 22-1, "IBLCE Examination Summary Data, 1985 – 1997." Based on the information provided, offer a brief overview characterizing the certification outcomes for the entire group of certification candidates.

4. Identify which health care providers should work together to assist the lactating mother of a breastfeeding baby who has failed to regain birth weight at one month of age. Explain how each person can provide assistance and in what ways they need to communicate with one another to effect optimal care in both the short - and the long - term.

5. You are asked by a student how one becomes a lactation consultant. Identify at least three sources of education this person might seek. Indicate why you recommend consideration of these educational offerings and how she might also gain direct hands-on supervision/mentoring in the local community.

6. Review Box 22-2 "Sample Time Expended to Provide LC Services in a Hospital," in the text. How closely does it match the experiences of LCs working in your local hospital? In what ways might the time spent by the local LC be changed if
   a. another LC is hired?
   b. the previous LC who assisted the current LC leaves her position?
   c. the hospital is merged with a local institution ten miles away?

7. Read the discussions of one 24-hour period on an Internet service relating to breastfeeding (if you are not connected to such a service, seek help from a colleague who is). What does review of these topics tell you about the concerns of LCs today?

Story Problem

You are a lactation consultant new to the town.

1. Indicate your credentials, if any, where your practice is located, and how you introduced yourself to both the health care community and the community at large.

You see the president of the local medical society one evening. He turns away from you with a scowl on his face.

2. What do you do? Why?

Later that week, you receive a letter indicating that your application for hospital privileges has been turned down.

3. What do you do? Why?

You've been working as a lactation consultant for three months. The two medical practices whose clients you serve as a prenatal breastfeeding educator have expanded. You are having difficulty meeting the needs of their pregnant clients and seeing them postpartum.

4. What three alternatives do you suggest to the physicians in these two practices? Why?

Three years have passed. At last night's medical staff meeting of the largest pediatric clinic in town–a practice you have served since your arrival–you receive a standing ovation for your tireless work with their clients. The founding member of the clinic hands you a bouquet of red roses and kisses you on the cheek.

5. How do you respond when the chief of service–who was vocally against your position–stands up to your applause, and states, "I always <u>knew</u> it was a good idea to hire her!"

CHAPTER

23

RESEARCH AND BREASTFEEDING

Outline

Key Concepts

You are urged to look for these key concepts in the body of the chapter and to develop questions deriving from these concepts as one way to gain understanding and insight into their relationship to lactation and breastfeeding. In this chapter, pay attention to the issues relating to the use of breastfeeding babies, lactating mothers, and human milk samples in a wide variety of research endeavors. When considering a research question, ask yourself whether sufficient attention has been paid to avoiding intrusion into the breastfeeding relationship – so that maternal milk production and/or infant behavior at the breast is not compromised. You may find that a careful review of these chapter elements highlights the many research questions that need to be asked – and that can be answered without harming the relationship you are seeking to understand more clearly.

Data analysis

Data collection

Ethnography

Grounded theory

Hypotheses

Methodology

Operational definitions

Phenomenology

Population

Quantitative and qualitative approaches

Reliability

Research problem, purpose

Review of literature

Rights of human subjects

Sampling

Setting

Validity

Variables

Multiple-Choice Questions

1. Grounded theory refers to a method
   a. used to understand beliefs, practices, and behavior patterns within the context of a particular culture or subculture.
   b. that focuses attention on those behaviors occurring on dirt floors.
   c. that generates a theory explaining an action within a particular social context.
   d. designed to understand the meaning of life experiences from the perspective of those who are living the experience under study.

2. An experimental study requires careful control of
   a. the first ten members of the first subject group.
   b. the totality of the subject groups.
   c. only those subjects randomized to the experimental group.
   d. only those variables considered to be independent to the experiment.

3. The variable that changes the action of a dependent variable is a(n)
   a. quasi-dependent variable.
   b. interventionist variable.
   c. independent variable.
   d. superior variable.

4. When a researcher chooses to write a null hypothesis, this means that
   a. the relationship between the dependent and independent variables is found to be null and void upon testing.
   b. the statement is written to predict no difference in the dependent variable by the action of the independent variable.
   c. the statement is written to predict a significant difference in the dependent variable only if at least two intervening variables also change.
   d. the relationship between the dependent and the independent variables is secondary to the relationship between the independent variable and at least two confounding variables.

5. Triangulation refers to
   a. the simultaneous use of multiple approaches to study a given phenomenon.
   b. the study of triangular devices in the collection of experimental data.
   c. the study of mother's nipples where the tissue comes to three points rather than a single point.
   d. the use of multiple approaches in a given order with a maximum of three methods.

6. The protection of human subjects derives from
   a. the actions of individuals who found that consent increased patient compliance in research protocols.
   b. the findings of studies first done on nonhuman primates which was subsequently attempted on human subjects.
   c. the requests of research subjects who insisted upon certain rights.
   d. the disclosure of inhumane acts that occurred during World War II.

Short-Answer Questions

1. Briefly define and distinguish between qualitative and quantitative research methods. Provide one example of a research question appropriate to each approach.

2. Briefly distinguish between descriptive, correlational, and experimental studies. Give an example of a research question appropriate to each type of study.

3. What is a quasi-experimental study?

4. What is triangulation? When might it be used? How might triangulation be used to strengthen the findings of a research study?

5. What is the importance of the rights of human subjects in a research study? How are these rights protected if the subject in question is
   a. the lactating mother?
   b. the breastfeeding baby?
   c. milk samples from several lactating mothers?

6. Briefly distinguish between a dependent and an independent variable.

7. What is an operational definition? Give an example.

8. Briefly distinguish between the purpose of a review of literature for a qualitative study and a review of literature for a quantitative study.

9. What is the difference between probability and nonprobability sampling? Give an example of each.

10. What is the difference between reliability and validity? Why is each important?

11. Describe phenomenology, ethnography, and grounded theory.

12. Provide an example of each of the following:
    a. descriptive method
    b. correlational method
    c. quasi-experimental method
    d. experimental method

13. Give an example of each of the following:
    a. observational question
    b. historical question
    c. feminist question

14. Define and give an example of each:
    a. dependent variable
    b. independent variable
    c. confounding variable(s)
    d. hypothesis

15. According to Katchum (1997), "breastfeeding duration was longest when the mother had previously breastfed, had a full-term baby, and was married; however, parity also showed a trend the opposite direction." Match each example in the right-hand column with the appropriate item in the left-hand column.
    a. dependent/outcome variable   1. marital status
    b. independent variable   2. parity
    c. confounding variable   3. previous breastfeeding experience
                                           4. breastfeeding duration
                                           5. full-term infant

16. Review one study that compares
    a. any breastfeeding with no breastfeeding.
    b. exclusive breastfeeding with two or more different feeding groups.
    Compare how the findings from each study can be
    c. generalized to the larger population.
    d. generate additional research questions (give 2 examples).
    Finally, explain why you would choose one study finding over the others, and relate this to the feeding definitions used.

17. Define and give an example of
    a. study setting.
    b. study population.
    c. study sample.
    d. sampling plan.

18. Distinguish between probability and nonprobability sampling, and give two different examples of each.

19. Review and compare interviews, field observations, and document review as alternative forms of data collection. What are the strengths of each? When might they be used? avoided? Give an example of a time when you, as a research investigator, might use each method.

20. Review interrater, intrarater, and test-retest reliability, and internal consistency. Give an example of each as you distinguish each from the other.

21. What is _____ validity? Give an illustrative example of each.
    a. concurrent
    b. construct
    c. content

Essay Questions

1. What elements are part of a quantitative method? In what sense are such methods considered "objective"?

2. What are the four basic rights of human subjects as determined by the Nuremberg Code? How might each relate to a study involving lactating mothers and/or their breastfeeding infants?

3. Distinguish among simple random sampling, systematic sampling, stratified random sampling, a sample of convenience, snowball sampling, and solicited sampling. Which is considered the most rigorous? Why?

4. Indicate when each of the following data collection techniques might be used. Give an example of a research question relating to breastfeeding which would be amenable to each technique.
    a. self-report questionnaire
    b. interview (face-to-face or telephone)
    c. observation (both when the subject is aware of the observation and when the subject is not)
    d. biophysiological measurement

5. In what ways might you determine that a research report is relevant to your work as a clinician?

6. How might researchers and clinicians work together to increase the likelihood that the research questions being posed are relevant to clinicians and the answers deriving from research endeavors can be used by clinicians?

Story Problem

You've been asked to design a study relating to lactation.

1. What research question have you decided to ask?

2. What is the research problem underlying the research question?

3. Who/what will serve as your research subjects?

4. What is the purpose of the study?

5. In what ways do you think this study will help other research investigators, as well as lactation consultants and other health care workers in clinical practice?

6. Outline the elements you would include in a consent form for this study.

7. What kind of sampling would you need to do?

8. What is your sample population?

9. How would you obtain your sample population?

10. If you plan to compare two or more groups, how do you distinguish between each group so that they are truly "discrete"?

11. How will you determine the reliability of the data you collect? its validity? its internal consistency?

12. What kinds of statistics will you use to analyze the data you've collected?

13. What is your <u>most important</u> finding? What two other findings will you discuss?

14. Indicate how the findings identified in question 13 could be used by clinicians working with breastfeeding mothers and babies in both an outpatient and a hospital setting. In what ways might these findings also generate additional research?

CHAPTER 24

Donor Human Milk Banking: More Than Nutrition

Outline

The history of human milk banking

Current trends in the United States and Canada

Donor-milk banking in countries outside North America

Cultural issues

The benefits of donor milk

Species specificity

Ease of digestion

Promotion of growth, maturation, and development of organ systems

Allergy prophylaxis

Immunological benefits

Clinical uses of donor milk

Distribution of donor milk: Neonates versus the older infants

Nutrition

Nutrition and disease prevention for premature infants

Milk fortification

Medicinal therapy

Current practice

Donor selection and screening

Heat treatment

Collection, handling, and storage

Packaging and transport

Quality assurance

Environmental contaminants

Policies and procedures

Costs of donor milk

Key Concepts

You are urged to look for these key concepts in the body of the chapter and to develop questions deriving from these concepts as one way to gain understanding and insight into their relationship to lactation and breastfeeding. In this chapter, you should pay attention not only to the history of human milk banking and its implications for product use today, but also to current concerns relating to donor selection, screening, handling of the milk, and quality assurance – and how human milk banking is likely to change in an era of heightened fear of bacterial and viral pandemics.

Banked human milk

Cultural issues

Donors of human milk

Environmental pollutants

Heat treatment

Marketing banked human milk

Milk collection

Milk handling

Milk screening

Milk storage

Quality assurance procedures

Multiple-Choice Questions

1. Human milk banks are a product of the
   a. late twentieth century.
   b. late nineteenth century.
   c. early twentieth century.
   d. late eighteenth century.

2. Bacteriological screening of raw human milk has revealed that
   a. premature infants are at risk when fed banked human milk.
   b. infants fed raw milk may receive high levels of coagulase-negative staphylococci.
   c. risk of sepsis from raw human milk feeds is very high.
   d. freezing is better than pasteurization for killing pathogens in human milk.

3. The number of milk banks throughout the world has declined over the past decade as a result of
   a. lack of interest by pediatricians.
   b. concern about transmitting HIV infections.
   c. concern about transmitting childhood diseases.
   d. lack of interest by tertiary health care centers.

4. Pasteurization of human milk is most likely to affect
   a. immunoglobulins.
   b. vitamins.
   c. live cells.
   d. bile salt-stimulated lipase (BSSL).

5. With the reunification of Germany, the number of milk banks in
   a. formerly East Germany climbed dramatically.
   b. formerly West Germany climbed dramatically.
   c formerly East Germany declined dramatically.
   d. formerly West Germany declined dramatically.

6. Holder pasteurization is
   a. milk held at 42.5°F for 30 minutes.
   b. milk held at 42.5°F for 60 minutes.
   c. milk held at 62.5°F for 30 minutes.
   d. no longer recommended as the standard method for pasteurization of human milk.

7. Which of the following practices is NOT part of the recruitment of human milk donors?
   a. heat treatment of all donated milk
   b. screening for health history and risk factors
   c. serological screening for certain viruses
   d. prevention of donation by mothers of babies who have died

Short-Answer Questions

1. Briefly explain why describing breastmilk as a form of altered blood may not be viewed as appropriate.

2. What is a graft versus a host reaction? How does it relate to donor milk?

3. Briefly explain why most banked milk is stored in pooled batches.

4. What do the FDA and CDC recommend regarding the heat treatment of banked human milk? Why is this important?

5. Briefly explain what lactoengineering is and how it might affect banked human milk.

6. What is quality assurance, and how is it incorporated into human milk bank procedures?

7. Briefly explain why environmental contamination is an issue for human milk banks.

8. What is a "kitchen" milk bank, and how might it be at risk for continued operation?

9. Explain the role of the Human Milk Banking Association of North America in establishing and maintaining a milk bank.

10. Describe how cultural beliefs can support or reduce the likelihood of using or donating milk for another mother's baby. Give at least one example to support your answer.

11. What is drip milk, and why is it less appropriate as a donation than actively expressed milk?

Essay Questions

1. Explain when donor milk might be used in a neonatal intensive care unit. Why is this not a universal practice in all NICUs?

2. What is the relationship between necrotizing enterocolitis, IgA deficiency, malabsorption syndrome, severe burns, inborn errors of metabolism, and banked human milk feedings?

3. How do each of the following affect banked human milk?
   a. heat treatment
   b. freezing
   c. handling
   d. packaging

4. Identify at least eight conditions for excluding potential breastmilk donors from offering their milk to a milk bank. Indicate whether each would be temporary or permanent.

5. Review how the distribution of banked milk has changed over time. Speculate on why this change has occurred.

Story Problem

You've been asked to provide instructions to a mother who wishes to donate her milk to a milk bank at her local hospital.

1. What do you tell this mother after she informs you that the hospital milk bank representative is out sick and that the donor mother has been asked to provide milk tomorrow?

2. Explain to the mother at least seven different situations in which her milk may be used.

The mother calls you and is indignant that she has been asked questions about HIV risk factors.

3. What do you tell her?

A local newspaper calls to ask for an interview about human milk banking in the era of AIDS.

4. How do you reply to the reporter's insistence on viewing human milk as a "carrier" of HIV?

A client from your practice is unable to totally nourish her baby on breastmilk following an auto accident in which she sustained injuries requiring extensive surgery on her upper chest. Her baby has responded poorly to all artificial baby milks offered. Your client asks if banked human milk, which the baby's pediatric gastroenterologist has suggested trying, is safe to use.

5. What is your reply?

6. What do you explain to her about how the milk is treated and what its effects might be on her baby?

The baby is now thriving; however, her intake is such that the milk bank coordinator is concerned about how long the local bank can continue to supply milk.

7. What do you suggest to the mother?

ANSWERS TO MULTIPLE-CHOICE QUESTIONS

Chapter 1
1. c
2. d
3. a
4. c
5. a
6. c
7. d
8. a

Chapter 2
1. d
2. a
3. d
4. b
5. a
6. d

Chapter 3
1. c
2. a
3. b
4. a
5. c
6. d
7. c

Chapter 4
1. b
2. a
3. b
4. b
5. d
6. d
7. b
8. c
9. d
10. a

Chapter 5
1. a
2. b
3. a
4. b
5. c
6. d
7. d
8. b
9. d
10. d
11. b
12. d
13. d
14. a
15. b

Chapter 6
1. a
2. d
3. d
4. b
5. b
6. c
7. d
8. b

Chapter 7
1. b
2. d
3. c
4. a
5. c
6. d
7. b
8. a

Chap. 8
1. d
2. a
3. c
4. d
5. c
6. a
7. d

Chapter 9
1. a
2. c
3. d
4. c
5. d
6. a
7. b
8. c
9. a
10. d

Chapter 10
1. c
2. d
3. b
4. d
5. b
6. a
7. b
8. a
9. c
10. b
11. d

Chapter 11
1. a
2. c
3. c
4. d
5. a
6. d
7. b
8. a
9. b
10. b

Chapter 12
1. b
2. c
3. b
4. b
5. a
6. a
7. b
8. a
9. d
10. a

Chapter 13
1. a
2. b
3. a
4. c
5. b
6. c
7. d
8. c
9. a

Chapter 14
1. d
2. b
3. c
4. d
5. a
6. c
7. d
8. b
9. c

Chapter 15
1. c
2. a
3. c
4. a
5. c
6. d
7. d
8. b
9. b
10. a

Chapter 16
1. a
2. d
3. b
4. c
5. a
6. c
7. d

Chapter 17
1. b
2. c
3. a
4. c
5. b
6. c
7. a
8. d

Chapter 18
1. c
2. b
3. b
4. d
5. d
6. a

Chapter 19
1. c
2. a
3. b
4. b
5. c
6. a

Chapter 20
1. a
2. c
3. d
4. a
5. b
6. a
7. b

Chapter 21
1. b
2. c
3. b
4. b
5. b
6. c
7. a

Chapter 22
1. a
2. c
3. a
4. c
5. a
6. d
7. c

Chapter 23
1. c
2. b
3. c
4. b
5. a
6. d

Chapter 24
1. c
2. b
3. b
4. b
5. c
6. c
7. d

STUDY QUESTIONS FOR APPENDICES TO *BREASTFEEDING AND HUMAN LACTATION*

Appendix A: Composition of Human Milk and Mature Breastmilk

1. A pregnant mother tells you that she very much wants to breastfeed but was told that colostrum has far fewer calories than does mature milk. She says the person who told her this also suggested that her first child's failure to gain weight adequately was because her milk was mostly colostrum and not "the real thing." How do you reply to this mother's concerns?

2. How important to the baby's growth and development is the absence of certain trace elements in colostrum?

3. A mother tells you that she is using megavitamins to boost what her two month-old baby will get from her milk. The vitamins she is taking in large quantities include vitamin A, vitamin D, riboflavin, vitamin B_6, and vitamin B_{12}. Which of these vitamins is likely to increase in the mother's milk? What do you tell her about the effect of taking megavitamins in this manner?

Appendix B: Via Christi Health System, St. Joseph Campus Breastfeeding Policies

1. Your hospital has adopted the Via Christi Health System, St. Joseph Campus Breastfeeding Policies. However, the original chairman of the Breastfeeding Policies and Protocols Committee, an individual who was instrumental in getting the policies adopted, has been replaced. The new chairman is an individual who never was supportive of such a change. Provide a justification for each of the 17 policies to convince the new chairman that the policies should stand.

2. Select one technique by which health care providers at your institution will make a functional assessment of the infant at the breast.
   a. Identify <u>why</u> you have selected this particular technique.
   b. Explain <u>how</u> you will teach this technique to staff nurses and house physicians who work with mothers and babies.
   c. Indicate <u>how</u> you will determine if this functional assessment
      (1) identifies babies and mothers in need of additional assistance.
      (2) identifies babies who are "nipple-confused."
   d. Explain <u>how</u> you will go about sharing what you have learned regarding this assessment technique with colleagues in your profession and other health care workers who assist breast-feeding mothers and babies.

3. Justify to a nurse manager why breastfeeding assessments require an average of 20 minutes - in a setting where nurse staffing has been severely eroded at the same time that your community has experienced a "birthing boomlet."

4. Explain how you would use a lactation consultant in a hospital where every nurse working with new mothers and babies has successfully completed a week-long training course designed to make them effective "lactation initiators."*

---

*S. S. Humenick: "A call for the lactation initiator: Setting the standards" (editorial), *J Hum Lact* 8:121, 1992.

5. Compare the breastfeeding policies from St. Joseph Medical Center and the Wellstart Lactation Program in San Diego. Identify similar individual policies from each set and compare them.
    a. How does each differ from the other? For example; how many times should a baby be offered the breast according to the St. Joseph policy? How does this relate to the recommendation pertaining to feeding frequency found in the Wellstart policy?
    b. Which differences suggest a need to rewrite that particular policy? If so, how would you recommend that it be rewritten, and why do you make this recommendation?
    c. Both policies provide supportive documentation for each of the policy statements. How would you support the selection of references? What criticisms might be offered?

Appendix C: Via Christi Health System, St. Joseph Campus Breastfeeding Education

An international evaluator of your maternity services is touring your unit and notes that you have developed the same breastfeeding education protocol that St. Joseph Medical Center uses. This visitor has several questions. Please provide a rebuttal to each of the following objections raised to the use of this protocol:

1. "Research has shown that undecided mothers are unimpressed with the benefits of human milk for babies as a reason for breastfeeding. Why do you bother with such information?"

2. "Your government gives away formula to poor mothers; therefore, the cost savings of breastfeeding is rendered moot. Why do you bother mentioning this as a benefit?"

3. "How can you say breastfeeding is 'convenient' when such a high proportion of new mothers in your city go back to work within a few weeks of their baby's birth? Surely, for them, bottle-feeding would be easier – if only because someone else can take responsibility for feeding the baby."

4. "If the mother can always change her mind and discontinue breastfeeding, aren't you admitting that modern formulas and breastmilk are equivalent and equally nutritious for the human infant?"

5. "You're very short-staffed. Why is it necessary for the nurse to take valuable time with each patient when you have all of these patient education materials she can take home?"

6. "At our hospital, 'kangaroo care' is practiced routinely in the NICU for as many babies as possible, including many who are less than 36 weeks gestation. We've found that these infants go to breast quite readily, often well in advance of 36 weeks. Given your insistence that breastfeeding is so much better for term babies, aren't you contradicting yourself by not offering preterms the same opportunity to breastfeed – simply on the basis of their gestational age?"

7. "You seem to have many 'rules' for optimal breastfeeding. Why don't you simply stand back, with your hands in your pockets, and watch how mothers and babies do it without help?"

8. "Technology seems to be highly valued in the United States. What would you do if you didn't have those extremely expensive, fancy breast pumps?"

9. "Please tell me how you know that a lactating breast is 'empty.' I'm unfamiliar with this concept."

10. "You don't seem to like mothers to supplement; however, many women do so, and your food stores and other places seem to stock all manner of artificial feeding gadgets. Don't you think you're fighting a losing battle?"

11. "You place great importance on mothers getting rest, but babies need to eat, often on a schedule unrelated to others' needs. How can you provide for the mother's need to rest and at the same time see to it that the baby gets to breast when he or she is most receptive to suckling?"

12. "I've noticed that on other floors in the hospital – including pediatrics – gifts don't go home with the patients. However, on the maternity floor, much is made of the opportunity for the hospital to give the mothers and babies something, as if such a gift will make them recall their experience more positively. Why do you think new mothers need such gifts?"

13. "Your answer to my previous question was very interesting. In my country, these 'gift packs' are simply not allowed in the hospital. Why don't you do that here?"

Appendix D: Nursing Diagnosis Related to Breastfeeding

Examine the definitions for effective breastfeeding, ineffective breastfeeding, and interrupted breast-feeding.

1. How would you incorporate these definitions and their respective defining characteristics into documenting/charting breastfeeding in a hospital or clinic setting?

2. In what ways might you improve on each of these definitions?

3. In what ways might these definitions be influenced by the cultural/ethnic group to which the mothers you assist belong?

Appendix E: New York State Code in Support of Breastfeeding (Added 1984)

1. How would you go about getting this code adopted in your state or province?
   a. Whom would you approach first, next? Why would you choose these individuals?
   b. In what ways might the breastfeeding mothers in your state or province get involved in such an action plan?
   c. How might your professional associations get involved?
      (1) Which groups are these?
      (2) What kind of role might each take?
   d. How might knowledge of breastfeeding initiation and duration rates be helpful in your campaign to get a code in support of breastfeeding adopted in your state or province?
   e. What about differences in breastfeeding initiation and duration by maternal ethnic/racial group, socioeconomic status, and other social factors?
   f. How might such a code benefit the hospitals or maternity centers in your state or province?

2. Are any hospitals in your state or province identified as "baby-friendly"? How might such a code assist a hospital in your community in reaching a goal of baby-friendliness?

3. How might such a state– or province–wide code assist in improving the care for breastfeeding mothers that currently characterizes the teaching centers in your state or province?

Appendix F: American Academy of Pediatrics: Breastfeeding and the Use of Human Milk

Review the AAP statement on breastfeeding and the use of human milk.

1. Identify at least seven different identified needs for breastfeeding, noting which pertain to a reduction in risk for the infant and for the mother.

2. What are the costs of not breastfeeding in one year? How does this relate to weekly and monthly costs of purchasing artificial baby milk for the individual family? How accurate is it for the costs in your community? Compare those costs with other costs likely to be incurred by a family in the same time period.

3. What barriers to breastfeeding initiation and duration are identified in this statement?

4. For each of the 12 recommended practices, note the following:
   a. Is this recommendation being put into practice in the local hospital or pediatric/family practice offices in your community?
   b. If it is not, how might you assist in its implementation as the standard of care?

Appendix G: Prototype Lactation Consultant Job Proposal or Description

1. Describe your own job as a lactation consultant in a hospital or clinic. If you have a private practice, describe the services you offer clients.

2. In what ways does your job description support the need for such a service in your community?

3. If you work in a hospital, how does what you do before the mother is discharged assist her past the first week of her newborn's life?

4. In what ways does your job description include coordinating your services with those of other health care professionals in the hospital and in the community? If it does not, how might you alter your practice to provide such a link between the services you offer and those available from others?

5. In what ways do you participate in scholarly activities, such as reading the professional literature, engaging in research studies, and writing grant proposals?
   a. How might you increase the frequency with which you engage in one or more of these activities?
   b. How would this activity help you in your practice?

6. In what ways do you participate in programs for the public or for other professionals about lactation and breastfeeding?
   a. How might you increase the frequency with which you engage in these activities?
   b. How would this activity help you in your practice?

Appendix H: ILCA Standards of Practice for Lactation Consultants

1. How might you use such a document to encourage the development of a lactation consultant service in a local medical center or clinic?

2. How might you use such a document to highlight the services you provide as a lactation consultant?

3. In what ways could you increase your own competency through a review of the competencies listed in the text of Appendix H?

4. How might elements noted in this document, but absent in your current LC job description, be used to enhance your proposal for an expansion of services with the addition of two more lactation consultants for your LC service?

Appendix I: Tables of Equivalencies and Methods of Conversion

1. Explain how you would use this table of equivalents in your daily practice. Why are such equivalents and conversion methods important to clinical practice?

2. Do you have a method of checking equivalents when working with a mother? What method or technique do you use? Why?

Appendix J: Wellstart International Patient History

1. Evaluate this patient history form.
   a. What are its strengths?
   b. In what ways do you feel it might be improved?
   c. How conveniently is it structured for clinical use?
   d. What elements might you add? Why?

2. What portions of this patient history would you be least likely to use? Why?

3. What portions of this patient history would you be most likely to use? Why?

Appendix K: Conversion Tables

1. Do you use such tables in your practice now? Why or why not?

2. When might such conversion tables come in handy?

3. Convert the following measures.

   10 gm = ____ ounces
   8 oz = ____ grams

   2 in = ____ centimeters
   12 cm = ____ inches

2 qt   =   ___ liters
4 L   =   ___ quarts (or ___ pints) (or ___ cups)
3 cups =   ___ ml

52°F   =   ___ °C
112°C   =   ___ °F

Appendix L: Standardized Height and Weight Growth Charts

An infant boy is seen in your office. Birth weight was 2590 grams, length was 18 inches.
  At three weeks, the baby weighs 3400 grams; length is 19.5 inches.
  At five weeks, the baby weighs 3480 grams; length is 20 inches.
  At seven weeks, the baby weighs 3520 grams; length is 20.25 inches.
  At eight weeks, the baby weighs 3550 grams; length is 20.5 inches.

1. Charting this infant's growth on the height and weight charts tells you what about the infant's pattern?

2. What suggestions will you offer to the mother and to the baby's primary care provider?

An infant girl is seen in your office. Birth weight was 3566 grams, length was 21 inches.
  At two weeks, the baby weighs 3700 grams; length is 21.25 inches.
  At four weeks, the baby weighs 4000 grams; length is 21.50 inches.
  At six weeks, the baby weighs 5000 grams; length is 22.25 inches.
  At eight weeks, the baby weighs 6800 grams; length is 22.50 inches.

3. After charting this baby's height and weight, what information do you share with the mother about her baby's growth?

4. What suggestions will you offer to the mother and to the baby's primary care provider?

GLOSSARY

Acinus Smallest division of a gland; a group of secretory cells arrayed around a central cavity. In the breast, an acinus secretes milk. Acini (pl). *See also* alveolus.

Aerobic Requiring air for metabolic processes (e.g., aerobic bacteria). Normal skin, including the breast, is colonized with aerobic bacteria.

Afferent Being conducted toward an organ or gland. Suckling produces afferent impulses which travel from the nipple to the pituitary gland, which then incites oxytocin release, causing milk to let down. The opposite of *efferent*.

Allergen Any substance causing an allergic response. Foods, drugs, or inhalants may be allergens. Cow's milk protein is a common allergen of infants.

Allopathic medicine A form of medical care characterized by a focus on the cure of disease presenting in a given organ or organ system; also called *Western medicine;* nonallopathic medicine is sometimes called *traditional* or *folk medicine* to distinguish it from the allopathic form.

Alphalactalbumin The principal protein found in the whey portion of human milk; it assists the synthesis of lactose. The dominant whey protein in cow's milk and most artificial infant milks, betalactoglobulin, is not found in human milk. *See also* Noncasein protein.

Alveolar ridge The ridge on the hard palate immediately behind the upper gums. Movement of the infant's jaw during nursing compresses the areola between his tongue and alveolar ridge.

Alveolus In the mammary gland, a small sac at the terminus of a lobule in which milk is secreted and stored. Alveoli (pl). Groups of alveoli, organized in lobes, give the mammary gland the appearance of a "bunch of grapes." *See also* Acinus.

Ampulla A normally dilated portion of a duct. Ampullae (pl). Ampullae in the lactiferous ducts underlie the areola near the base of the nipple. *See also* Lactiferous sinuses.

Anorectal abnormalities Anomalies of the rectum, the lower few inches of the large intestine, and the anus, the opening in the skin at the distal end of the rectum. An example is imperforate anus, in which the rectum ends in a blind pouch.

Antibody An immunoglobulin formed in re-sponse to an antigen, including bacteria and viruses. Antibodies then recognize and attack those bacteria or viruses, thus helping the body resist infection. Breastmilk contains antibodies to antigens to which either the mother or the infant has been exposed.

Antigen A substance that stimulates antibody production. It may be introduced into the body (as dust, food, or bacteria) or produced within it (as a by-product toxin).

Antigenemia The state of having an antigen of interest in the blood.

Applied research Research that focuses on solving or finding an answer to a clinical or practical problem.

Areola Pigmented skin surrounding the nipple that overlies the ampullae or lactiferous sinuses. In order to suckle effectively, an infant should have his gums placed well back on the areola.

Artificial infant milk Any milk preparation, other than human milk, intended to be the sole nourishment of human infants.

Atopic eczema An inherited allergic tendency to rashes or inflammation of the skin. Exclusively breastfed infants are less likely to manifest this condition, as cow's-milk protein is a common allergen.

Atresia, intestinal Congenital blockage or closure of any part of the intestinal tract.

Axilla The underarm area; in it lies the uppermost extent of the mammary ridge or milk line. Deep breast tissue (the axillary tail or tail of Spence) extends toward and sometimes into the axilla. This tissue may engorge the axilla along with the rest of the breast in the early postpartum period.

B cell A lymphocyte produced in bone marrow and peripheral lymphoid tissue and is found in breastmilk. It attacks antigens and is one type of cell that confers cell-mediated immunity.

Bactericidal Capable of destroying bacteria. Breastmilk contains so many bactericidal cells that the bacteria count of expressed milk actually declines during the first 36 hours following milk expression.

Bacteriostatic Capable of inhibiting the proliferation of bacterial colonies.

BALT/GALT/MALT Bronchus/gut/mammary-associated immunocompetent lymphoid tissue. A lymphocyte pathway that causes IgA antibodies to be produced in the mammary gland after a lactating woman is exposed to an antigen on her intestinal or respiratory mucosa. These antibodies are then transferred through breastmilk to the breastfeeding infant, who thus may possess antibodies to antigens to which he has not been directly exposed.

Banked human milk *See* Donor milk.

Basic research Research that generates knowledge for the sake of knowledge.

Betalactoglobulin The dominant protein present in the whey fraction of the milk of cows and other ruminants; it is absent from human milk.

Bias Any factor, action, or influence that distorts the results of a study.

Bioavailable That portion of an ingested nutrient actually absorbed and used by the body. Because the nutrients in breastmilk are highly bioavailable, low concentrations may actually result in more nutrients being absorbed by the infant than do the higher, less bioavailable concentrations in cow's milk or artificial infant milks.

Bivariate Statistics derived from the analysis of the relationship between two variables.

Buccal pads Fat pads sheathed by the masseter muscles in young infants' cheeks. The buccal pads touch and provide stability for the tongue, which enhances the tongue's ability to compress breast tissue during suckling. Breastfed infants typically have a plump-cheeked appearance because of well- developed buccal pads.

Candidiasis A fungal infection caused by *Candida albicans;* also called "thrush." Common in the maternal vagina, it may inoculate the infant during delivery and be transferred from the infant's mouth to the mother's nipple. Candidiasis of the nipple and breast may produce intense nipple and breast pain. In the infant, it may produce white spots on the oral mucosa and a bright red, painful rash ringing the anus. Formerly termed moniliasis.

Casein The principal protein in milks of all mammals. Human milk has a ratio of soluble whey proteins to casein of about 65:35. Casein of human milk forms soft, easily digested curds in the infant stomach. The whey-to-casein ratio in cow's milk is 20:80; artificial infant milks have whey-to-casein ratios that vary from those of cow's milk to 40:60. Cow's-milk casein forms firm curds that require a high expenditure of energy to digest.

Centers for Disease Control (CDC) An agency of the U.S. Public Health Service established in 1973 to protect the public health of the nation by providing leadership and direction in the prevention and control of diseases and other preventable health conditions, and to respond to public health emergencies.

Certification The process by which a nongovernmental professional association attests that an individual has met certain standards specified by the association for the practice of that profession.

Chi-square A statistical procedure that uses nominal level data and determines significant differences between observed frequencies in relation to the data and expected frequencies.

Colostrum The fluid in the breast at the end of pregnancy and in the early postpartum period. It is thicker and yellower than mature milk, reflecting a higher content of proteins, many of which are immunoglobulins. It is also higher in fat-soluble vitamins (including A, E, and K) and some minerals (including sodium and zinc).

Concept A word, idea, or phenomenon that generally has abstract meaning.

Conceptual framework A structure of interrelated concepts that may be generated inductively by qualitative research or provide a base for a quantitative study.

Congenital infection An infection existing at birth that was acquired transplacentally. Infections that may be so acquired include HIV and TORCH organisms. *See also* Human immunodeficiency virus; TORCH.

Conjunctivitis Inflammation of the mucous membrane that lines the eyelid. In many traditional and some modern societies, fresh breastmilk is instilled into the eyes to alleviate this condition.

Construct A cluster of several concepts that has abstract meaning.

Contraception Preventing conception. Breast-feeding provides significant contraceptive protection during the first few months postpartum–as long as the infant is fully breastfed and feeds during the night, and maternal menses have not resumed.

Cooper's ligaments Triangular, vertical ligaments in the breast that attach deeper layers of subcutaneous tissue to the skin.

Cord blood Blood remaining in the umbilical cord after birth.

Correlation coefficient A statistic that indicates the degree of relationship between two variables. The range in value is +1.00 to –1.00; 0.0 indicates no relationship, +1.00 is a perfect positive relationship, and 1.00 is a perfect inverse relationship.

Creamatocrit The proportion of cream in a milk sample, determined by measuring the depth of the cream layer in a centrifuged sample. An indicator of caloric content of milk, which must be used with care; the fat (and thus caloric) content of human milk varies between breasts, within a feeding, diurnally, and over the entire course of lactation.

Cross-nursing Occasional wet-nursing on an informal, short-term basis, usually in the context of child care.

Cultural relativism Recognition of the wide variation in beliefs and actions that pertain to given behaviors in different cultures.

Culture The values, beliefs, norms, and related practices of a given group that are learned and shared by the group members and that guide both the thoughts and behaviors of that group.

Cytoprotective Any condition or factor that protects cells from inflammation or death.

Deductive reasoning The process of reasoning from a general premise to the concrete and specific.

Dependent variable The variable the investigator measures in response to the independent or treatment variable; the outcome variable that is affected by the independent variable.

Design The blueprint or plan for conducting a study.

Diagnostic-related grouping (DRG) A group of diagnoses for health conditions that result in similar intensity of hospital care and similar length of hospital stay for patients hospitalized with those conditions.

Diffusion The process by which the molecules of one substance (e.g., a drug) are spread uniformly throughout a given substance (e.g., blood or plasma). *Passive diffusion* refers to movement from a higher to a lower concentration; *active diffusion* refers to movement from a lower to a higher concentration.

Disaccharide A carbohydrate composed of two monosaccharides. The principal sugar in human milk is lactose, a disaccharide; its constituent monosaccharides are glucose and galactose.

Donor milk Human milk voluntarily contributed to a human milk bank by women unrelated to the recipient.

Donor milk, fresh-frozen Fresh-raw milk that has been stored frozen at –20°C for less than 12 months.

Donor milk, fresh-raw Milk stored continuously at 4°C for not longer than 72 hours after collection.

Donor milk, heat-treated Fresh-raw milk or fresh-frozen milk that has been heated to a minimum of 56°C for 30 minutes.

Donor milk, pooled A batch of milk containing milk from more than one donor.

Dopamine The prolactin-inhibiting factor (PIF), or a mediator of PIF, secreted in the hypothalamus. It blocks the release of prolactin into the bloodstream.

Drip milk Milk that leaks from a breast that is not being directly stimulated. Because its fat content is low, this milk should not be used regularly for infant feedings.

Ductules Small ducts in the mammary gland that drain milk from the alveoli into larger lactiferous ducts that terminate in the nipple.

Dyad A pair (e.g., the breastfeeding mother and her infant).

Eczema Skin inflammation or rash. *See also* Atopic eczema.

Elemental formula Artificial infant milks containing fats, proteins, and carbohydrates in their simplest (most elemental) forms.

Eminences of the pars villosa Tiny swellings on the inner surfaces of infant's lips that help the infant to retain a grasp on the breast during suckling.

Energy density The number of calories per unit volume; caloric density. Mature human milk averages 65 calories/dl, controlled largely by the fat content of the milk.

Envelope virus A virus that cannot infect other cells without its coat (envelope). If the envelope is destroyed (e.g., by heat or soap and water), the ability of the virus to produce infection is destroyed. Cytomegalovirus and the human immunodeficiency virus are envelope viruses.

Epidemiology The study of the frequency and distribution of disease and the factors causing that frequency and distribution.

Epiglottis Cartilaginous structure of the larynx. An infant's epiglottis lies just below the soft palate. It closes the larynx when the infant swallows, ensuring passage of milk to the esophagus.

Estrogen A hormone that causes growth of mammary tissue during part of each menstrual cycle and assists in the secretion of prolactin during pregnancy; one of the hormones whose concentration falls sharply at parturition.

Ethnocentrism A view that one's own culture and how it defines appropriate behavior is used as the basis for assessing all other cultures and behaviors.

Ethnography One research method that attempts to support an understanding of the beliefs, practices, and behavioral patterns within a (sub)culture from the perspective of the people living in that culture.

Exogenous Derived from outside the body–e.g., iron supplements that provide the infant with exogenous iron.

External validity The extent to which study findings can be generalized to samples different from those studied.

Extraneous variable Variables that can affect the relationship of the independent and dependent variables, i.e., interfere with the effect of treatment. In experimental studies, strategies for controlling these variables are built into the research design.

Foremilk The milk obtained at the beginning of a breastfeeding. Its higher water content keeps the infant hydrated and supplies water-soluble vitamins and proteins. Its fat content (1–2 gm/dl) is lower than that of hindmilk.

Frenulum Fold of mucous membrane, midline on the underside of the tongue, that helps to anchor the tongue to the floor of the mouth. A short or inelastic frenulum, or one attached close to the tip of the tongue, may restrict tongue extension enough to inhibit effective breastfeeding. Called also the frenum.

Fructose A carbohydrate present in small quantities in human milk.

Galactagogue Any food or group of foods thought to possess qualities that increase the volume or quality of milk produced by the lactating woman who eats such foods.

Galactopoiesis The maintenance of established milk synthesis that is controlled by the autocrine system of supply and demand.

Galactorrhea Abnormal production of milk. It may occur under psychological influences or be a sign of pituitary tumor.

Galactose A monosaccharide present in small quantities in human milk. It is derived from lactose and, in turn, helps to produce elements essential for the development of the human central nervous system.

Gastroenteritis Inflammation of the stomach and intestines resulting from bacterial or viral invasion. Breastfed infants are at lower risk for this illness, as compared to nonbreastfed infants.

Gastroschisis An opening in the wall of the abdomen; a congenital malformation.

Gestational age An infant's age since conception, usually specified in weeks. Counted from the first day of the last normal menstrual period.

Half-life The length of time for half of a drug dosage to be eliminated; generally, it takes four to five half-lives for a drug to be considered completely or nearly completely eliminated. *Example:* Half-life of drug A is 12 hours, so 50 percent of the original drug dosage is eliminated in 12 hours; 25 percent of the drug is remaining after 24 hours; 12.5 percent of the original dosage is remaining after 36 hours; 6.25 percent of the original dosage is present after 48 hours, and only 3.12 percent is present after 60 hours (five half-lives from time of original dosage).

Hindmilk Milk released near the end of a breastfeeding, after active let-down of milk. Fat content of hindmilk may rise to 6 percent or more, two or three times the concentration in foremilk.

Horizontal transmission Transmission of pathogens through direct contact. *See also* Vertical transmission.

Human immunodeficiency virus (HIV) A retrovirus that disarms the body's immune system, causing death from an opportunistic infection. First identified in 1981. The virus may be transmitted to unborn infants, and it is carried in the breastmilk, although not all breastfed infants born to HIV-positive mothers become ill themselves. The greatest risk to the infant is posed when a woman experiences her initial HIV-related illness while pregnant or breastfeeding.

Human milk Milk secreted in the human breast.

Human milk bank A service that collects, screens, processes, stores, and distributes donated human milk to meet the needs of those, usually infants, for whom human milk has been prescribed by a physician.

Human milk fortifiers Nutrients added to expressed human milk to enhance the growth and nutrient balances of very low-birth-weight infants. Added protein may be derived from protein components of donor human milk or from cow's-milk-based products. *See also* Lactoengineering.

Hydration The water balance within a body. Adequate hydration is necessary to maintain normal body temperature and for most other metabolic functions. Breastmilk is 90 percent water. Therefore, even in hot or dry climates, a fully breastfed infant obtains all the water he requires through breastmilk.

Hyperalimentation The intravenous feeding of an infant, commonly a very premature infant, with a solution of amino acids, glucose, electrolytes, and vitamins.

Hyperosmolar A fluid that is of higher osmotic pressure than the reference fluid. Elemental formulas are hyperosmolar; breastmilk is isoosmolar with human serum.

Hyperprolactinemia Higher-than-normal prolactin levels, which may result in spontaneous breastmilk production and amenorrhea. Causes include pituitary tumors and some pharmaceuticals. *See also* Prolactin.

Hypothalamus A gland that controls postpartum serum prolactin levels through release of dopamine. Inhibition of dopamine permits the release of prolactin, which controls the secretion of milk.

Immunity, active Immunity conferred by the production of antibodies by one's own immune system.

Immunity, passive Immunity conferred on an infant by antibodies manufactured by the mother and passed to the infant transplacentally or in breastmilk. Passive immunity is temporary but very important to the young infant.

Immunoassay Any method for the quantitative determination of chemical substances that uses the highly specific binding between antigen or hapten and homologous antibodies (e.g., radioimmuno-assay, enzyme immunoassay, and fluoroimmunoassay).

Immunogen A substance that stimulates the body to form antibodies. *See also* Antigen.

Immunoglobulin Proteins produced by plasma cells in response to an immunogen. The five types are IgG, IgA, IgM, IgE, and IgD. IgG is transferred in utero and provides passive immunity to infections to which the mother is immune; IgA is the principal immunoglobulin in colostrum and mature milk; IgM is produced by the neonate soon after birth and is also contained in breastmilk. *See also* Noncasein protein.

Incidence How much a particular behavior is practiced at a given time. *Example:* How many women are initiating breastfeeding from time A to time B?

Incubation period The period between exposure to infectious pathogens and the first signs of illness.

Independent variable The experimental or treatment variable that is manipulated by the investigator to influence the dependent variable.

Inductive reasoning The process of reasoning from specific observations or abstractions to a general premise.

Infection control Practices–in hospitals formalized by protocols–that reduce the chance that infection will be spread between patients or between patients and staff. Hand washing and wearing of rubber gloves are two such practices.

Internal validity The extent to which manipulation of the independent variable really makes a significant difference on the dependent variable rather than on extraneous variables.

International Code of Marketing of Breast-Milk Substitutes A set of resolutions that regu-late the marketing and distribution of any fluid intended to replace breastmilk, certain devices used to feed such fluids, and the role of health care workers who advise on infant feeding. Developed by members of a joint commission convened in 1979 by WHO and UNICEF, it was approved in 1981 by members of the WHO (only the United States dissented). Intended as a voluntary model that could be incorporated into the legal code of individual nations in order to enhance national efforts to promote breastfeeding. Also referred to as the *WHO Code* or the *WHO/UNICEF Code.*

Intracellular Occurring within cells. Viruses live within other cells during part of their reproductive lives. Although virus within cells may be passed to the infant in breastmilk, other cells in breastmilk enhance the destruction of these infected cells.

Intrauterine Within the uterus; in utero.

Intrauterine growth rate The normal rate of weight gain of a fetus. It is considered by many, but not all, physicians to be the ideal growth rate for premature infants.

Involution Refers to the return of the mammary gland to a nonproductive state of milk secretion.

Lactase Enzyme needed to convert lactose to simple sugars usable by the infant. Present from birth in the intestinal mucosa, its activity diminishes after weaning.

Lactase deficiency *See* Lactose intolerance.

Lactiferous ducts Milk ducts; 15 to 24 tubes that collect milk from the smaller ductules and carry it to the nipple. They appear similar to stems on a bunch of grapes, the alveoli being the "grapes." The ducts open into nipple pores.

Lactiferous sinuses Dilations in the lactiferous ducts under the areola that act as small milk reservoirs. To nurse effectively, an infant must take enough breast into his mouth to be able to strip milk from these sinuses.

Lactobacillus bifidus Principal bacillus in the intestinal flora of breastfed infants. Low intestinal pH (5–6) of fully breastfed infants discourages the colonization of *Streptococcus faecalis, Bacteroides sp.* and *E. coli,* which are common in feces of infants fed cow's-milk-based infant milks.

Lactoengineering The process of fortifying human milk with nutrients (especially protein, calcium, and phosphorus) derived from other batches of human milk, in order to meet the special nutritional needs of very low-birth-weight infants. *See also* Human milk fortifiers.

Lactoferrin A protein that is an important immuno-logical component of human milk. It binds iron in the intestinal tract, thus denying it to bacteria that require iron to survive. Exogenous iron may upset this balance. *See also* Noncasein protein.

Lactogenesis The initiation of milk secretion. The initial synthesis of milk components that begins late in pregnancy may be termed *lactogenesis I;* the onset of copious milk production two or three days postpartum may be termed *lactogenesis II.*

Lactose The principal carbohydrate in human milk; about 4 percent of colostrum and 7 percent of mature milk. A disaccharide, it metabolizes readily to glucose, which is used for energy, and galactose, which assists lipids that are laid down in the brain. Lactose also enhances calcium absorption, thus helping prevent rickets in the breastfed infant, and it inhibits the growth of pathogens in the breastfed infant's intestine.

Lactose intolerance   The manifestation of lactase deficiency; the inability of the intestines to digest lactose, the principal carbohydrate in human milk. More common beyond early childhood because of diminished activity of intestinal lactase, especially in cultures that do not use milk or milk products as foods after early childhood.

Larynx   The region at the upper end of the trachea (windpipe) through which the voice is produced. In the infant, the larynx lies close to the base of the tongue; during swallowing, it rises and is closed off by the epiglottis.

Lesion   Circumscribed area of injured or diseased skin.

Let-down   The milk-ejection reflex. Caused by contraction of myoepithelial cells surrounding the alveoli in which milk is secreted. It is under the control of oxytocin released during nipple stimulation and, sometimes, of psychological influences.

Leukocytes   Living cells, including macro-phages and lymphocytes, that inhabit breastmilk and combat infection.

Licensure   The process by which an agency of state government grants permission to an individual, who is accountable for the practice of a profession, to engage in that profession. The corollary of licensure is that unlicensed individuals are prohibited from legally practicing licensed professions. The purpose of licensure is to protect the public by ensuring professional competence.

Ligand   A small molecule that binds specifically to a larger molecule (e.g., the binding of an antigen to an antibody, or of a hormone to a receptor).

Likert scale   A scale that primarily measures attitudes by asking respondents their degree of agreement or disagreement for a number of statements.

Lipase   Enzyme that aids in the digestion of milk fats by reducing them to a fine emulsion.

Low-birth-weight   Term applied to infants weighing less than 2,500 gm at birth.

Lymphadenopathy   Abnormal swelling of lymph nodes.

Lymphocyte   A mature leukocyte; a lymph cell that is bactericidal.

Lyophilization   A process of rapid freeze-drying of a fluid under a high vacuum. This process is used on human milk to obtain nutrient fractions used to fortify expressed human milk.

Lysozyme   Enzyme in breastmilk that is active against *Escherichia coli* and *Salmonella. See also* Noncasein protein.

Mammary bud   A clump of embryonic epithelial cells formed along the mammary ridge that extend into the underlying mesenchyme. It develops about 49 days postconception. From this bud sprout the precursors of the milk ducts.

Mammary ridge   Milk line; the linear thickening of epithelial cells to each side of the midline of the embryo. Develops during weeks 5 through 8. Later this ridge differentiates into breast and nipple tissue.

Mammogenesis   The development of the mammary gland and related structures within the breast.

Mandible   The lower jaw. Strong, rhythmic closing of the mandible during breastfeeding drives the compression of the lacteriferous sinuses, one component of the infant's milking process.

Mature milk   Breastmilk commonly produced after about two weeks postpartum and containing no admixture of colostrum. It is higher in lactose, fat, and water-soluble vitamins. Its exact composition varies in response to infant needs.

Median   The middle number in a series of numbers; the number on either side of which exist an equal amount of numbers.

Mesenchyme   The embryonic mesoderm.

Milk-plasma ratio   The quantity of a given drug or its metabolite in human milk in relation to its quantity in the maternal plasma or blood. Gen-erally, if the M/P ratio exceeds 1.00, the drug is found in lesser quantities in milk than in plasma. If the M/P ratio is less than 1.00, the drug is found in lower quantities in milk than in plasma.

Mitosis   A type of cell division in which each daughter cell contains the same DNA as the parent cell.

Morbidity   The number of ill persons or instances of a disease in a specific population.

Mortality   The number of deaths in a specific population.

Mucocutaneous   Involving both mucous membranes and skin. Herpes blisters, for example, can form on both sites.

Multiparous   Having carried two or more pregnancies to viability.

Myelination   The process by which conducting nerve fibers develop a protective fatty sheath. The long-chain polyunsaturated fats that are important to myelination are abundant in human milk; they are much less abundant in cow's milk or cow's-milk-based infant milks. Loss of myelin is a characteristic of the disease multiple sclerosis.

Myoepithelial cells Contractile cells. In the breast, these cells surround the milk-secreting alveoli; their contraction forces milk into the milk ducts. When many of these cells contract at the same time, a let-down occurs. *See also* Let-down.

Necrotizing enterocolitis Inflammation of the intestinal tract that may cause tissue to die. Premature infants not receiving human milk are at markedly greater risk for this serious complication of premature birth.

Neurotransmitter A chemical that is selectively released from a nerve terminal by an action potential and then interacts with a specific receptor on an adjacent structure to produce a specific physiologic response.

Nipple Cylindrical pigmented protuberance on the breast into which the lactiferous ducts open. The human nipple contains 15 to 20 nipple pores through which milk flows. The mammary papilla.

Nipple, inverted A nipple that is retracted into the breast both when at rest and when stimulated.

Noncasein protein The protein in the whey portion of milk. Noncasein proteins in human milk include alphalactalbumin, serum albumin, lactoferrin, immunoglobulins, and lysozyme.

Nongovernmental organization (NGO) Title conferred by UNICEF on private organizations that command expertise valuable to UNICEF; such organizations are permitted to comment on and attempt to influence UNICEF activities. La Leche League International and the International Lacta-tion Consultant Association are NGOs.

Nonparametric statistics Statistical procedures used when required assumptions for using parametric procedures are not met.

Nonprotein nitrogen (NPN) About one-fourth of the total nitrogen in human milk is derived from sources, such as urea, other than protein. NPN contains several free amino acids, including leucine, valine, and threonine, which are essential in the young infant's diet because he cannot yet manufacture them.

Nutriment Any nourishing substance.

Oligosaccharide Carbohydrate, comprised of a few monosaccharides, present in human milk. Some oligosaccharides promote the growth of *Lactobacillus bifidus,* thus increasing intestinal acidity, which discourages the growth of intestinal pathogens.

Operational definition Explicit description of a concept or variable of interest in measurable terms.

Oral rehydration therapy (ORT) The administration by mouth of a solution of water, salt, and sugar in order to replace body fluids lost during severe diarrhea. The proportions of elements in an oral rehydration solution are essentially the same as they are in breast-milk. Artificially fed infants are much more susceptible than those who are breastfed to the diarrhea that may lead to severe dehyration and the need for ORT.

Oxytocin A lactogenic hormone produced in the posterior pituitary gland. It is released during suckling (or other nipple stimulation) and causes ejection of milk as well as uterine contractions.

Palate, hard The hard, anterior roof of the mouth. A suckling infant uses his tongue to compress breast tissue against the hard palate.

Palate, soft The soft, posterior roof of the mouth, which lies between the hard palate and the throat. It rises during swallowing to close off nasal passages. Also called the velum.

Parametric statistics Statistical procedures used when a sample is randomly selected, represents a normal distribution of the target population, and is considered sufficiently large in size and interval level data are collected.

Parenchyma The functional parts of an organ. In the breast, the parenchyma include the mammary ducts, lobes, and alveoli.

Parenteral Introduction of fluids, nutrients, or drugs into the body by any avenue other than the digestive tract.

Pasteurization The heating of milk to destroy pathogens. Milk banks commonly heat donor milk to 56° for 30 minutes.

Pathogen Substance or organism capable of producing illness.

Peristalsis Involuntary, rhythmic, wavelike action. Commonly thought of in relation to food and waste products moving along the gastrointestinal tract. In order to strip milk from the breast, an infant's tongue uses a peristaltic motion that begins at the tip of the tongue and progresses toward the back of the mouth.

Pharynx The muscular tube at the rear of the mouth, through which nasal air travels to the larynx and food from the mouth travels to the esophagus. During infant feeding, contraction of pharyngeal muscles moves a bolus of fluid into the esophagus.

Pituitary An endocrine gland at the base of the brain that secretes several hormones. Prolactin, which is essential for production of milk, is secreted by the anterior lobe; oxytocin, which is essential for milk let-down, is secreted by the posterior lobe.

Placenta   The intrauterine organ that transfers nutrients from the mother to the fetus. The expulsion of the placenta at birth causes an abrupt drop in estrogen and progesterone, which in turn permits the secretion of milk.

Polymastia   The presence of more than two breasts. These additional structures, which usually contain only a small amount of glandular tissue, may occur anywhere along the milk line from axilla to groin.

Population   The total set of individuals that meet the study criteria from which the sample is drawn and about whom findings can be generalized.

Power   The probability that a statistical test will reject a null hypothesis when it should be rejected, or in other words, detect a significant difference that does exist.

Premature infant   One born before 37 weeks' gestational age, regardless of birth weight.

Prevalence   How much a given behavior is occurring at a given time as well as how long that behavior is practiced. *Example:* the combined effect of breastfeeding initiation rates and breastfeeding continuance and duration rates.

Primary infection   The first incidence of illness after exposure to a pathogen.

Primiparous   Having carried one pregnancy to viability.

Progesterone   Hormone produced by the corpus luteum and placenta that maintains a pregnancy and helps develop the mammary alveoli.

Prolactin   Hormone that is produced in the anterior pituitary gland. It stimulates development of the breast and controls milk synthesis. Normal concentrations are 10–25 ng/ml in a nonpregnant woman; 200–400 ng/ml at birth.

Prone   Lying on one's stomach.

Reliability   The degree to which collected data are accurate, consistent, precise, and stable over time.

Respiratory syncytial virus (RSV)   Organism causing a respiratory illness; breastfed infants are at less risk for this illness than are nonbreastfed infants.

Rickets   Abnormal calcification of the bones and changes in growth plates that lead to soft or weak bones. Rarely seen in breastfed children; exceptions include those not exposed to the sun.

Rotavirus   A class of viruses that are a major cause of diarrheal illness leading to hospitalization of infants. Breastfed infants are at less risk for illness caused by this organism, as compared to breastfed infants.

Rugae   Corrugations on the hard palate behind the gum ridge that help the infant to retain a grasp on the breast during suckling.

Sample   A subset of the population selected for study.

Sampling   The procedure of selecting the sample from the population of interest.

Sebaceous glands   Glands that secrete oil. Those on the areola are called the *tubercles of Montgomery;* the oil they secrete is presumed to lubricate and provide bacteriostatic protection to the areola.

Secretory IgA   An immunoglobulin abundant in human milk that is of immense value to the neonate. It is synthesized and stored in the breast; after ingestion by the infant, it blocks adhesion of pathogens to the intestinal mucosa.

Secretory immune system   The system that produces specific antibodies or thymus-influenced lymphocytes in response to specific antigens.

Sepsis   The presence of bacteria in fluid or tissue.

Seroconvert   A process by which serum comes to show the presence of a factor that previously has been absent, or vice versa. When antibodies to an infecting agent, such as cytomegalovirus, become present the person is said to have seroconverted.

Serological tests   Tests performed on blood samples to ascertain the presence or absence of pathogens.

Seronegative   Serum that does not demonstrate the presence of a factor for which tests were conducted; "tests negative."

Seropositive   Serum that demonstrates the presence of a factor for which tests were conducted; "test positive."

Serum   Clear fluid portion of blood that remains after coagulation.

Serum albumin   A protein in serum. *See also* Noncasein protein.

Smooth muscle   The type of muscle that provides the erectile tissue in the nipple and areola.

Somatic   Pertaining to the body, especially nonreproductive tissue.

Spontaneous lactation   Secretion and release of milk unrelated to a pregnancy or to nipple stimulation intended to stimulate milk production.

Suck, Suckle   Used in this textbook interchangeably to mean the baby's milking action at the breast. In traditional usage, a baby at the breast "sucked," whereas a mother "suckled."

Sucking, nonnutritive   Sucking not at the breast (e.g., as on a pacifier or on baby's own tongue); or sucking at the breast characterized by alternating brief sucks and long rest periods during minimal milk flow. However, insofar as any milk is transferred, even this latter pattern of sucking may, in fact, be nutritive. *See also* Sucking, nutritive.

Sucking, nutritive Steady rhythmic sucking during full, continuous milk flow. Insofar as any milk is transferred, other sucking patterns also may be nutritive. *See also* Sucking, nonnutritive.

Supine Lying on one's back.

Symbiosis The intimate association of two different kinds of organisms. The breastfeeding dyad is considered by many to exemplify a mutually beneficial symbiosis.

Systemic immune system The nonspecific immune responses of the body.

T cells Any of several kinds of thymic lymphoid cells or lymphocytes that help to regulate cellular immune response. A subset of these cells (T_4 cells) are preferentially attacked by the human immunodeficiency virus.

Target population The population that is of interest to the investigator and about which generalizations of study results are intended.

Teleological Describing the belief that all events are directed toward some ultimate purpose.

Thrombocytopenia Low levels of platelets in blood.

TORCH Acronym for organisms that can damage the fetus: toxoplasmosis, rubella, cytome-galovirus, herpes simplex.

Tracheoesophageal fistula (T-E fistula) An abnormal opening between the trachea and esophagus; this congenital malformation occurs in about 1 in 3,000 births. T-E fistula may cause a neonate to aspirate fluids. Colostrum, a physiologic fluid, is much less irritating to the lungs than water, glucose water, or artificial infant milks.

Transcutaneous bilimeter A device that estimates bilirubin concentrations in the blood by measuring intensity of yellowish skin coloration.

Transitional milk Breast fluid of continuously varying composition produced in the first two to three weeks postpartum as colostrum decreases and milk production increases.

Transplacental Transferred from mother to fetus through the placenta. Nutrients and certain immunoglobulins are, and some infections may also be, transferred to the fetus transplacentally.

United Nations Children's Fund (UNICEF) Originally established in 1946 as the United Nations International Children's Emergency Fund. An agency of the United Nations charged with protecting the lives of children and enabling children to lead fuller lives. It assists member nations in providing health care, safe water, sanitation, nutrition, housing, education, and training to accomplish these goals.

Univariate Statistics derived from analysis of a single variable, e.g., frequencies.

Universal precautions Guidelines for infection control based on the assumption that every person receiving health care carries an infection that can be transmitted by blood, body fluids, or genital secretions.

Vaccine An infectious agent, or derivatives of one, given to a person so that his or her immune system will produce antibodies to that infection without a preceding illness.

Validity The degree to which collected data are true and represent reality; the extent to which a measuring instrument reflects what it is intended to measure.

Variable Attributes, properties, and/or characteristics of persons, events, or objects that are examined in a study.

Vertical transmission Transmission of infection from mother to child transplacentally or through breastmilk.

Very low-birth-weight Term applied to infants weighing less than 1,500 gm at birth.

Virus Very small organisms that rely on material in invaded cells to reproduce. Viruses identified in breastmilk include cytomegalovirus, *herpes zoster, herpes simplex,* hepatitis, and rubella.

Water-soluble vitamins The B vitamins and vitamin C, pantothenic acid, biotin, and folate. These vitamins are present in serum; concentrations in breastmilk approximate those in serum. Concentrations reflect current maternal diet more directly than do fat-soluble vitamins (A, D, E, K).

Wet nurses Women who, for pay, breastfeed infants who are not their own.

Whey The liquid left after curds are separated from milk. Alphalactalbumin and lactoferrin are the principal whey proteins. Because human milk has a whey-to-casein ratio of about 65:35, it forms soft, easily digested curds in the infant stomach. *See also* Casein, Noncasein protein.

Witch's milk Colostrum, formed under the influence of maternal hormones, which may be expressed from temporarily enlarged mammary tissue in the neonate's breasts.

World Health Organization (WHO) An agency of the United Nations charged with planning and coordinating global health care and assisting member nations to combat disease and train health care workers.

Xerophthalmia Disease of the eyes caused by vitamin A deficiency; endemic in parts of Africa. Human milk is a preventive.

MEDICAL ABBREVIATIONS USED THROUGHOUT
BREASTFEEDING AND HUMAN LACTATION

>	greater than
<	less than
=	equal to
ā	before
ab	abortion
ABC	alternative birthing center
abd	abdomen
ABG	arterial blood gases
AIDS	acquired immunodeficiency syndrome
BBT	basal body temperature
Bf	breastfed/breastfeeding
BMD	bone mineral density
B/P	blood pressure
BPD	bronchopulmonary dysplasia
BSE	breast self-examination
BUN	blood urea nitrogen
C	centigrade
c̄	with
CA	cancer
Ca	calcium
cal	calorie
CHD	congenital heart disease
CBC	complete blood count
cc	cubic centimeter
CMV	cytomegalovirus
CNM	certified nurse midwife
CNS	central nervous system
CPAP	continuous positive airway pressure
C&S	culture and sensitivity
c/sec	cesarean birth
CSF	cerebral spinal fluid
CVA	cardiovascular accident
CVP	central venous pressure

D5W	5% dextrose in water
D&C	dilation and curettage
D/C	discharge
dc	discontinue
DR	delivery room
DRG	diagnostic related groups
dx	diagnosis
ECG	electrocardiogram
EDC	estimated date of confinement (due date)
EDD	estimated date of delivery
EEG	electroencephalogram
EENT	eyes, ears, nose, throat
EFM	electronic fetal monitoring
epis	episiotomy
ER	emergency room
ET	endotracheal tube
FAS	fetal alcohol syndrome
FBD	fibrocystic breast disease
FBS	fasting blood sugar
FLK	funny-looking kid
FSH	follicular stimulating hormone
FTT	failure to thrive
FUO	fever of unknown origin
GDM	gestational diabetes mellitus
GI	gastrointestinal
gm	gram
gr	grain
grav	gravida (number of pregnancies)
GU	genitourinary
GYN	gynecology
hct	hematocrit
Hg	mercury
H&P	history and physical
ht	height
hx	history

IDDM	Insulin-dependent diabetes mellitus	pH	degree of acidity/alkalinity
IUGR	intrauterine growth retardation	PID	pelvic inflammatory disease
IM	intramuscular	PIH	pregnancy-induced hypertension
I&O	intake and output	PKU	phenylketonuria
IUD	intrauterine device	po	by mouth
IV	intravenous	prn	as needed
		PT	physical therapist
JCAH	Joint Commission on the Accreditation of Hospitals	q	every, each
		qd	every day
Kg	kilogram	qid	4 times/day
L	liter	Ⓡ	right
Ⓛ	left	RBC	red blood cell
lab	laboratory	RDA	recommended dietary allowances
LC	lactation consultant	RDS	respiratory distress syndrome
LGA	large for gestational age	REM	rapid eye movement
LMP	last menstrual period	Rh	Rhesus blood factor
		R/O	rule out
Mcg	microgram	Rx	medication/prescription
mec	meconium		
med	medication	s̄	without
mg	milligram	SGA	small for gestational age
ml	milliliter	SIDS	sudden infant death syndrome
		SOAP	subjective data, objective data, analysis, plan
NANDA	North American Nursing Diagnosis Association	staph	staphylococcus
NEC	necrotizing enterocolitis	STD	sexually transmitted disease
n/g	nasogastric	strep	streptococcus
NPO	nothing by mouth		
NSAID	nonsteroidal anti-inflammatory drug	tid	3 times/day
nsg	nursing (breastfeeding)		
		u/a	urinalysis
Ø	no, none	URI	upper respiratory infection
OB	obstetrical	UTI	urinary tract infection
OT	occupational therapy		
OTC	over the counter	VBAC	vaginal birth after cesarean
oz	ounce		
		WBC	white blood cell
p̄	after	WIC	Special Supplemental Food Program for Women, Infants, and Children
para	number of living children		
pc	after meals (post cibum)		
PCR	polymerase chain reaction		
PDA	patent ductus arteriosus		
peri	perineal		